THE
POWER
OF
GOD'S WORD

FOR
HEALTHY LIVING

VOLUME 4

A CHRISTIAN DEVOTIONAL
WITH PRAYERS FOR HEALING
AND SCRIPTURES FOR HEALING

BY ANNE B. BUCHANAN

The Power of God's Word for Healthy Living: A Christian Devotional with Prayers for Healing and Scriptures for Healing (Christian Devotional Healing Series, Volume 4) Copyright © 2011, 2014, 2018 by Anne B. Buchanan

Disclaimer / Limitations of Liability

All material in this book is for information and educational purposes only. No information concerning matters of health is intended as a means to diagnose or treat diseases. No information is intended to be a substitute for medical advice by a licensed health care provider. All readers should consult a licensed health care provider and The Great Physician in all matters relating to medical problems, especially in matters of diagnosing or treating diseases or other physical and mental conditions. The Author and Publisher do not directly or indirectly give medical advice, nor do they prescribe any supplements or assume any responsibility or liability for those who treat themselves. No statements in this publication have been analyzed or approved by the FDA.

Dedicated

To The Glory of God
Who Loves Us
And Who Heals Us

In Memory of
My mother, Elizabeth

TABLE OF CONTENTS

SECTION TWO
Good Nutrition for Healthy Living

SECTION THREE
Healthy Emotions for Healthy Living

SECTION FOUR
Spiritual Guidelines for Healthy Living

Great Resources

✝

PREFACE

This is Volume 4 in *The Power of God's Word* series of Christian devotionals on healing. God wants us to be well, and He wants us to act in partnership with Him to build habits of health in our lives. In this book we will explore numerous Scriptures that reveal God's messages to us on ways we can establish good habits for healthy living to strengthen our minds and our bodies.

I have divided this volume into four basic categories:
Section 1 – A Strong Body for Healthy Living
Section 2 – Good Nutrition for Healthy Living
Section 3 – Healthy Emotions for Healthy Living
Section 4 – Spiritual Guidelines for Healthy Living

Remember that the foundations for many of the Biblical principles that I discuss in these devotions are laid in *The Power of God's Word for Healing*, Volume 1 and *The Power of God's Word for Receiving Healing*, Volume 2.

In this book I assume from the beginning that you believe that it is God's will for you to be well. I also assume that you believe that Jesus took every sickness upon Himself and that by His stripes you are healed. If you are not in agreement or you have questions about these two principles, please refer to *The Power of God's Word for Healing*, Volume 1 and *The Power of God's Word for Receiving Healing*, Volume 2 for a thorough explanation.

In my own personal life, I find that God's Word and God's remedies make a powerful combination for healing. The God who created me also created the plants, herbs, and essential oils, and I believe He did so with full *intention* – knowing exactly how my body works and how these natural substances meet my bodily needs. However, I want to emphasize that I never forget that it is the Creator who is to be exalted, not the creation. It is the Lord God Almighty who is my Healer, rather than any substance which I may use temporarily to assist my bodily functions to return to a proper balance.

Each person has to take full responsibility for his own health and make his own personal decision about medical care. Those who are on medications need to be particularly cautious. Some medications create a serious physical dependency in the natural world and to discontinue them suddenly can lead to rapid death unless God intervenes supernaturally. God's Word tells us we are not to tempt Him.

Therefore, to discontinue any medication in a rush of "instant faith" would most likely be a fatal decision that would delight the evil one. Don't do it. Instead, strengthen your faith, pray with your medical counselors, and seek God's instruction and your doctor's instructions about what changes to make and when to make them. I am not a medical doctor and do not prescribe or suggest any medical treatments. Please heed the disclaimer at the beginning of this book and seek appropriate health care professionals in matters concerning your health.

Please note that I have occasionally taken a few liberties with the English language in this book. I have bent a few rules of grammar so that what you read matches the way that people speak. I have also intentionally spelled satan's name with a small "s" except at the beginning of a sentence. Writing his name in lower case provides a visual reminder that he has been totally defeated by our Risen Savior and has only the power we choose to give him.

This book proclaims God's healing power in small daily doses, boosting our faith step by step and reminding us of God's Holy Word and His covenant with us. It is easy to talk about faith and quite another to navigate the path of healing with focus and purpose. I hope that all who read these messages will be blessed by them.

At the end of the book are a few selected references to materials which you may find useful if you wish to explore further. I am very grateful for those who have long proclaimed God's healing message and who have been instrumental in helping me along the way.

If you like this volume of *The Power of God's Word*, please check out the other volumes in the series, which are available from Amazon .com in paperback and on Kindle. Audiobooks are available from Amazon.com, iTunes.com, and Audible.com.

We also have a YouTube channel called Proclaiming God's Word, which has uplifting, encouraging, and peaceful videos on topics such as Scriptures for healing,

Scriptures for sleep, and Scriptures for overcoming depression. Please take a look at them at:

http://YouTube.com/c/ProclaimingGodsWord.

Many blessings to each one of you,

Anne Buchanan

P.S. If you like this book, it would be a great blessing to me if you would go to Amazon.com and leave a review in the "Customer Reviews" section. Thank you.

SECTION ONE

A STRONG BODY FOR HEALTHY LIVING

What are the basic elements
involved in
building your body?

✝

DAY 1
BUILD YOUR BODY WITH WISDOM

Through wisdom is an house builded; and by understanding it is established: and by knowledge shall the chambers be filled with all precious and pleasant riches. (*Proverbs 24:3-4*)

When you have a health condition, one of the essential ingredients to being a partner with God for your healing is to seek knowledge about it. There are two major facets of learning for you to focus on.

The first concerns the way that your body works. The emphasis is not on the illness that has attacked you but on the function of a healthy body. By studying how the different systems of the body are supposed to work in unison and harmony with each other, you get a clear picture of what the word "health" should mean.

Once you know how a healthy body should be, look for common links between your various health conditions. For example, suppose your triglyceride level is high and your blood sugar level is at the high end of the normal range. In this case, one possible link is a malfunctioning pancreas.

The second aspect of study concerns God's remedies for human health problems. Since God designed your body, no human is ever likely to understand the way that it functions as thoroughly as He does. Do not forget that fact when you receive emphatic opinions, especially ones of doom from human beings.

When God created plants, He considered them to be so critical to the well-being of people that one of the two first instructions He gave to man was to order that they be used for food to nourish and strengthen our bodies. Therefore, search for God's remedies.

Remember Ezekiel's vision when he saw trees lining a river, "... and the fruit thereof shall be for meat [food], and the leaf thereof for medicine [healing]" (Ezekiel 47:12). Some of man's medicines are beneficial and useful, but to label God's remedies as inferior or old-fashioned or out-moded is pure folly. Scripture said long ago, "My people are destroyed for lack of knowledge" (Hosea 4:6).

Why are we so stubborn in refusing to allow God's leadership? Open your mind and heart to the glory of God's creation and to the use of God's remedies (essential oils and herbs) for your healing where you are guided to do so.

Almighty God, help me to build a strong temple for Your glory. Give me wisdom to seek Your advice and guidance for every step I take on my path to recovery. Show me the way to find books, teachers, and instruction so that I may expand my understanding of my body and Your remedies. Thank You for sending Your Son, who bore my illnesses on the Cross and who has redeemed me – spirit, soul, and body. In Jesus' name, I pray, Amen.

✝

DAY 2
YOU ARE WONDERFULLY MADE

I will praise thee; for I am fearfully and wonderfully made.
(Psalm 139:14)

How right David was! We are fearfully and wondrously made. We are awesome in spirit, soul, and body.

We can choose to believe the theory that we evolved to have the bodies we do, or we can choose to believe that God specifically designed our bodies to function according to His holy design. God's Word says that He created us as human beings. Our scientific knowledge has grown exponentially, yet what we do not know about the functioning of our bodies far exceeds what we do know.

God designed us to live. He put specific intelligence in each cell so that it can carry out its function and so that we do not have to give any thought to supervising each of these trillions of cells. Events occur externally or internally, and our trillions of cells respond. This happens every millisecond of every day of every year.

When we make wise choices and provide our bodies with positive experiences, we become partners with God in creating health. When we make foolish or destructive choices, we become partners with satan in creating illness. Satan works so stealthily that often it is only after months, years, and decades of seemingly inconsequential choices that we begin to manifest disease.

Perhaps we are too wondrously made! What would happen if we put sugar water in our car's gasoline tank? It wouldn't take thirty, forty, or fifty years for us to know we had violated the basic rules for the proper functioning of the car.

What would happen if we turned our vacuum cleaner on and kept it on for twenty hours every day, day after day after day? It wouldn't be able to hold up for twenty years being pushed like that, would it? Yet because our bodies are so wondrously made, we can often "get away" with violating God's rules for healthy eating, exercising, and resting for forty years before illness begins to manifest.

Who is your partner? Choose Jehovah-Rapha, the God who heals you. Make a decision to glorify Him by keeping your temple strong and healthy. Praise your Creator for making your body in such a wondrous way.

Father God, I praise You because I am, indeed, fearfully and wonderfully made. You created my spirit, soul, and body through Your mighty power, and I give You all the glory. I accept my responsibility for my health choices, and I choose to honor my body as the temple of the Holy Spirit. I will do everything I can to maintain its good health. I rejoice that I can proclaim Your Word as absolute truth. Jesus took my infirmities and bore my sicknesses. By His stripes I am healed. In Jesus' name, I pray, Amen.

†

DAY 3
OFFER YOUR BODY TO GOD

Therefore, I urge you, brothers, in view of God's mercy, to offer your bodies as living sacrifices, holy and pleasing to God – this is your spiritual act of worship. (Romans 12:1 New International Version)

Paul exhorts you to offer your body to God as a living sacrifice and as a spiritual act of worship. Would it make a difference in your choices if you thought of every movement of your body and every act you do for it and to it as an act of worship to the Lord God Almighty?

Most of the things we do are accomplished without much conscious thought at all. Our nose itches and we scratch it. Our muscle feels cramped and we stretch it. Our stomach growls and we eat. Our bodies feel ill and we reach for a drug. Rarely do we think of any of these things as an act of worship.

Whether you feel sick or whether you feel well, offer your body to God as a living sacrifice, holy and pleasing to Him. God is your Creator. He made you, and, therefore, your body is pleasing to Him as a reflection of His majesty and creative power. Your body was designed as a temple, the temple of the Holy Spirit. It is a magnificent instrument for God's purpose.

There is no human being who really understands how an egg and a sperm can unite, instantly forming a unique person, who in time will be composed of trillions of cells, each one filled with life, each one having a specific function, and each one fulfilling its purpose in harmony with the others. No one ever will. Scientists may dangerously experiment with cloning life that already exists, but it is the breath of God – and God alone – that *creates* life.

Because your body is God's holy creation, you should look to God for instruction on its care. Let God's Holy Word show you the proper nourishment and food for it. Let God guide you to the use of His own remedies through essential oils or herbs or to treatment by spirit-led medical personnel. Let God be your sole authority, and let everything you use regarding your health function as an instrument for working God's will.

God has breathed in you the breath of life and He wants you well. He wants you to glorify and worship Him with your body.

Heavenly Father, I offer my body to You as a living sacrifice. May it be holy and pleasing to You as Your awesome creation. I honor and respect my body and treat it lovingly and with care. I enforce Your Word upon it and declare that by the stripes of Jesus I am healed. Thank You, Father, for healing me. In the mighty name of Your Son, Christ Jesus, I pray, Amen.

✝

DAY 4
WE NEED GOD-GUIDED SCIENCE

*Know ye that the Lord he is God: it is he that hath made us, and
not we ourselves.   (Psalm 100:3)*

There is only one Creator of all life and that is God.
Our own creations are to be the result of revelation
knowledge and guidance from Him.   They are not to be
solely for material gain and power, but they are to make the
world better, safer, and healthier.   God always wants us to
act in partnership with Him rather than to work indepen-
dently in our own strength.

However, the very definition of science now excludes the
belief in or the relevance of God.   That leaves the scientific
community particularly susceptible to the influence of
satan, and, when we create under the influence of the evil
one, we sow the seeds of our own destruction.   It is a godless science that leads us to poison our foods with chemicals
and convinces us that there are no health consequences.

It is a godless science that genetically alters fruits and
vegetables into synthetic food that can sit on the shelf for
weeks without rotting and convinces us that there are no
health consequences.   It is a godless science that manipu-
lates plants so that they cannot produce seeds of their own
that will germinate and convinces us that there are no
health consequences for our children.   It is a godless science

that clones animals and convinces us that there are no health and spiritual consequences.

We need science, but we need a God-guided science. If you agree, do what you can to speak out and express your concerns. On the personal level, take full responsibility for your health. As much as possible, eat organic food that is grown as God intended the plant to be. You cannot live in divine health without having nourishing food.

Ask God to lead you to counselors and advisors (both medical and otherwise) who will pray with you and will be willing to consider both God-provided and man-made solutions to your health problems.

Almighty God, I declare that You and only You are the Great Creator. It is You who have made me and You alone. Help me always to seek Your advice as I choose my food and as I make decisions on treatments offered by science. I know that You want me to be well and that You will direct my path so that I can make the choices that are best for my recovery. In Jesus' name, I pray, Amen.

✝

DAY 5
LEARN HOW YOUR BODY WORKS

There is a way which seemeth right unto a man, but the end thereof are the ways of death.   (Proverbs 14:12)

We, as human beings have limited knowledge, wisdom, and understanding. Despite the fact that we actually know so little, we often forget we are not God. We declare science to be built on facts that are absolute and conveniently forget how over the years scientific "facts" have changed as our knowledge has changed. In *Confessions of a Medical Heretic*, Dr. Robert Mendelsohn writes that modern medicine is "neither an art nor a science" but that its foundation depends on patients' trust and faith in it.

Most people do not know that Hippocrates, the father of medicine, emphasized herbs and nutrition for his patients rather than medicines because he was concerned about their harmful effects. The statement, "Whenever a doctor cannot do good, he must be kept from doing harm," is attributed to him. He recognized that herbs are concentrated foods and nourish the body to help it overcome the basic problem of the illness.

We get off the track when we separate our learning from our belief in God. As we engage in scientific exploration, our endeavors should be in partnership with God and in agreement with God's will. When we pretend that God has no place in science, however, we become easily led by the enemy into reckless arrogance. What seems to be logical and "right," ultimately leads to death.

God gave us intelligence, and He wants us to learn about the human body so that we may help in the healing process when there is illness. There can be a time and place for drugs, surgery, and other medical treatments. However, we must be very careful when we alter God's design for life and health so that we do not find ourselves on a path leading to untimely death.

Look to God's herbs, essential oils, and healing substances, and learn about them. Then learn about the things that the mind of man has devised. But, first and foremost, pray for guidance, and follow the course God desires for you and your healing.

Almighty God, I pray for those scientists who are filled with Your Holy Spirit and who are working to benefit all people. When I have medical tests and am told that certain results will happen unless I have certain treatments, remind me, Father, to seek Your guidance after hearing these opinions. Help me to make my decisions based on Your truth rather than on my fear. Show me Your way and I will follow it. In Jesus' name, I pray, Amen.

✝
DAY 6
YOUR BODY IS A HOLY HABITATION

In whom ye also are builded together for an habitation of God through the Spirit.   (Ephesians 2:22)

You are the habitation of God because the Holy Spirit dwells in you. Since your body is the earthly vessel, the earthly home, of this precious Holy Spirit, it is your responsibility to take care of it. Your body is a holy temple and must be treated as such.

Pay attention to your body and treat it with care and kindness. How many things each day do you do to be kind to your body? How much time do you give to creating a healthy environment for your body?

Some actions are really simple and take only moments. For example, while you are working, take a minute – sixty little seconds – to stop and breathe deeply. You may choose to look at the sky or just close your eyes and inhale slowly and fully. As you do so, thank God for your life and for healing you – body and soul. Take one of these prayer moments every thirty minutes and see how vitalizing it can be.

Other things take more time and more commitment. Spending time exercising your body requires commitment, especially if you have a sedentary lifestyle.

Walking is perhaps the ideal exercise because it also allows you to renew yourself spiritually at the same time. While you are walking, notice nature around you, whether it is the sky above, a flower struggling through a crack in the sidewalk, or the trees that surround you. Find something each day, and say "thank You" to God.

Preparing healthy meals with as much organic produce as possible takes time, effort, and sometimes financial sacrifice. And another part of healing through nutrition is adding herbs to your diet. Check out some books about herbs from the library. Find a health food store where the people are knowledgeable.

Learn as much as you can about God's remedies because they are God's gifts to us. Honor your holy temple, and give it respect, attention, and loving care.

Dear God, You have given me this body as a precious temple of the Holy Spirit and as Your habitation. Help me to care for it with love, nourishing it physically and spiritually. Sometimes I feel too tired to do the things I know I should do. And sometimes I just seem too busy with the trivia of life. Remind me of Your priorities, Father, and keep me focused on the things that are truly important so that I can join in full partnership with You for my health. Thank You. In Jesus' name, I pray, Amen.

✝

DAY 7
ARE GERMS THE PROBLEM?

... Stand up and bless the Lord your God for ever and ever: and blessed be thy glorious name, which is exalted above all blessing and praise. Thou, even thou, art Lord alone; thou hast made heaven, the heaven of heavens, with all their host, the earth, and all things that are therein, the seas, and all that is therein, and thou preservest them all; and the host of heaven worshippeth thee. (Nehemiah 9:5-6)

The Lord God Jehovah gave life to everything. The heavens, the earth, you – and even some of the germs, bacteria, and viruses that we so love to hate. We can only speculate that the most dangerous "bugs" have mutated because of our fallen world. Certainly God did not create any organisms with the purpose of killing us.

We seem to spend our time focused on killing viruses and bacteria. Yet illness cannot take hold within us unless the environment exists for it to grow. Contrary to popular belief, disease is not due as much to the existence of germs in our bodies as it is to the fact that conditions in us are optimal for those germs to grow and multiply. For example, at this very moment you probably have the strep virus in your body, yet you probably do not have strep throat. Why? Because your immune system is working effectively to keep the strep virus from causing any problem for you. Most illnesses and diseases work that way.

During the Middle Ages a great plague swept Europe and killed over one-third of the population. What about the other two-thirds? The people who did not die were exposed to the same germs, but their immune systems had the strength to identify, resist, and destroy the invading bacteria.

Interestingly, a band of thieves went among the sick, dying, and dead, stealing objects of value from the bodies without ever getting the deadly plague. When they were captured, they were forced to reveal their secret. They had covered themselves with a blend of essential oils, including cloves, cinnamon, eucalyptus, and rosemary, that raised their immune levels so that they did not succumb to the disease.

Let your focus be on those things which give life. Learn how the systems of your body function, what nutrients you need to support those systems, which sources of those nutrients are best for you, and how you can strengthen all the parts of your body which are weak. Seek the Holy Spirit's counsel and then act on the guidance that is given to you.

Almighty God, You have made the heaven, the earth, all life, and me. Help me to glorify You by learning how I can strengthen my own body. Send me teachers, and I will learn. I promise to act on my knowledge, according to the guidance from the Holy Spirit. Thank You. In Jesus' name, I pray, Amen.

✝

DAY 8
THE DANGER OF BAD HABITS

Be well balanced (temperate, sober of mind), be vigilant and cautious at all times; for that enemy of yours, the devil, roams around like a lion roaring [in fierce hunger], seeking someone to seize upon and devour.   (1 Peter 5:8   Amplified Bible)

What a vivid picture this is of how the devil works! He stalks around like a lion on the prowl, looking for someone to seize and devour. If only he always came in the form of a lion, we probably wouldn't fall into his traps so easily. But he is usually a disguised lion and hopes to catch us unaware.

Sometimes satan seems to devour us in one big gulp, but usually he nibbles and nibbles and nibbles at us. He attacks us with fear and then uses it against us if we don't take control over it. He knows our most sensitive vulnerabilities and relentlessly exploits them.

He chips away at our health through one tiny decision after another. Just one order of French fries, even though we know they are filled with harmful grease. Just one more day with our feet up, even though we know our bodies need some exercise. Just one more night of staying up past midnight, even though we know our bodies need rest in order to heal. Just one more ...

The list goes on and on. One unhealthy decision will not harm us. But we have a way of forgetting how many of them we make.

What does Peter say we must do to avoid being caught by the devil? Be well balanced. Be vigilant. Be cautious. These recommendations are especially important when we feel sick, although they may seem harder to follow then because we may have less energy.

Stand firm against the enemy by taking the authority given to you in Luke 10:19. Bring people into your life who will support you, encourage you, and give you feedback to alert you when they see your vigilance waning. Have them join you in prayer to resist the evil one. Jesus paid the ultimate price for you to walk in triumph.

Accept your responsibility to take action and give God all the glory for your victory.

Father God, Your Word makes it clear that the devil has come to steal, kill, and destroy. He has attacked me and wants to take my health, my time, my money, and my joy. I repent for ways that I have opened the door to these attacks, and I now take my authority and bind every attack of the enemy in the name of Jesus. Thank You, Father, for the victory You have purchased for me through the blood of Your glorious Son, in whose name I pray, Amen.

✝

Day 9
The Challenges Of Using Healthy Light

Truly the light is sweet, and a pleasant thing it is for the eyes to behold the sun. (Ecclesiastes 11:7)

Light. The glory light. It was the first thing God created, and it was also the way Jesus described Himself. Then on day four of creation, the Lord God created the sun to bless us with its warmth and benefits. Light is essential both for our spirit and for a healthy body.

Light actually has healing properties. Through exposure to the sun, our bodies manufacture vitamin D. Unfortunately, many of us spend almost no time in the sun during the day, and our bodies consequently suffer from lack of exposure to God's natural light.

It is healthy to spend a minimum of twenty to forty minutes a day in the sunshine. Those people with abundant nutrient intake from their food rarely experience skin problems from reasonable exposure to the sun. Conventional medical advice requires people to use sunscreen, but among natural health professionals there is no current agreement whether the benefits actually outweigh the risks.

When indoors, we need to use the proper type of light. Until recently, most people used "regular" incandescent bulbs which emit light rays from only part of the full spectrum of the sun. The government has mandated that the manufacture of this type of bulb to cease, but they are promoting a much more detrimental type of lighting – fluorescent bulbs. This type of lighting saps your strength and your energy. It is damaging to health, and studies show that children exhibit more attention-deficit symptoms and hyperactivity when exposed to those lights.

The healthiest kind of light bulbs are incandescent full-spectrum bulbs. If you change the bulbs in your home and your workplace to full spectrum lighting, you will notice that your eyes do not become as fatigued and that your energy level increases. It is amazing the results we experience when we return to God's plan for our health instead of using artificial methods that are not in synchronization with the way that our bodies function. It is worth your time to do your own investigation and make up your own mind about the lighting that is healthiest for you to use in your home.

Jesus told us, "I am the light of the world" (John 9:5). He was speaking both of glory light and of natural light. If you are able to do so, go outside and stand in God's natural sunlight. Breathe deeply, glorifying your Heavenly Father with each breath and allowing the Lord's glory-light to fill you while His sunlight bathes your body. As the air fills your lungs, feel the light from the sun shining on you. Command every organ, gland, and cell in your body to receive God's light.

No matter what your situation is at this very moment, "let your light shine before men" (Matthew 5:16). Your faith is a great light that can be a beacon to others. In spite of any challenges you have, know that Jesus has won your victory – so shine, shine, shine.

God of Glory, I will take the time to enjoy Your sunshine in a wise and healthy manner, and I will provide healthy lighting for myself when I am indoors. I want to spend more time in the light of the sun outside and to spend more time in the light of the Son in my heart and soul. I want my light to shine before others so that they will come to praise You as I do. In the name of Jesus Christ, my Savior and my Redeemer, I pray, Amen.

✝

Day 10
Pure Water Is Essential
For Life

You make springs pour water into the ravines, so streams gush down from the mountains. They provide water for all the animals, and the wild donkeys quench their thirst. The birds nest beside the streams and sing among the branches of the trees. You send rain on the mountains from your heavenly home, and you fill the earth with the fruit of your labor. (Psalm 104:10-13 New Living Translation)

Water is essential for life. God has provided it in great abundance, both outside our bodies (the earth is about 70 percent water) and inside our bodies (we are about 65 percent water). Without sufficient water we can survive only a few days because the cells of the body cannot function properly without it. For example, water is critical in our eliminative process and in the regulation of our body temperature. Many illnesses come upon us after many years of partial dehydration of our bodies.

Think about the water described in this lovely Psalm and then consider what we do to water. We routinely dump waste materials into our water supply and then add more chemicals to attempt to clean it up enough to drink.

We add fluoride, which is a potent poison, on the erroneous assumption that it prevents cavities in teeth. The fluoride enters the long bones of our body and replaces calcium. This makes the bones rigid instead of flexible. So in our folly, we end up with brittle bones and with bone fracture rates 2-3 times as high as those people who drink unfluoridated water. This fact (as well as several other disturbing effects) is the reason that very few countries in the world still allow fluoride to be put in the water supply.

We also add chlorine to kill bacteria, which it does effectively. Unfortunately, however, studies as old as the 1930s show that chlorine is also linked to various types of heart disease, now the leading cause of death in our country.

Are these health problems God's will? Of course not. He plainly told us that He gave us dominion over the earth (Genesis 1:28). We are listening to the lies of the evil one, killing ourselves, and then blaming God for it.

In order for you to be healthy, it is vital to drink wholesome water. Whether it be distilled water with added minerals or pure spring water, find the healthiest supply you can. God will not be mocked. To be well you must return to the basics, and water is one of the most essential.

Almighty God, maker of heaven and earth, I seek to return to Your plan for life by consuming healthy water. I have taken water for granted and haven't made the effort to see that I drink and bathe in water that promotes my good health. I understand now how I have contributed to my health problems, and I return to Your plan for pure water. In Jesus' name, I pray, Amen.

✝

DAY 11
HOW TO BREATHE PROPERLY

And the Lord God formed man of the dust of the ground, and breathed into his nostrils the breath of life; and man became a living soul. (Genesis 2:7)

Every time we breathe, we affirm the moment of our creation. Of all bodily activities, breathing is one of the most essential. Few people can sustain life without breathing for more than three minutes or so. Ironically, most of us develop poor breathing habits that contribute to the improper functioning of our bodies.

Watch an infant while it is sleeping. Notice that the entire abdominal area rises with each inhalation and falls with each exhalation. Babies breathe naturally from their diaphragm, pulling the air deeply into the lungs. As children grow up, they encounter stressful events and gradually tighten various muscle groups. By adulthood, most of us breathe shallowly from the upper parts of our lungs.

Stop for a moment and take a deep breath. Did you raise your shoulders in the process? When your abdominal muscles and diaphragm are relaxed and your breathing habits are healthy, your abdomen extends as you inhale and your shoulders do not move. When your abdominal muscles are tight, your abdomen remains rigid and your

41

upper chest is pushed outward as the upper lungs fill with air. You are forced to raise your shoulders.

Every cell of your body desperately needs oxygen. Life cannot exist without it. There is evidence that there was a much higher concentration of oxygen in the air at the time of the creation of Adam and Eve, and the effect of our industrial and chemical pollution is to increase the depletion of this vital nutrient. Take responsibility in your own life to reduce the chemicals that you use that have a negative impact on your air, your environment, and your body.

Learn to breathe properly. One of the easiest ways to do this is to incorporate proper breathing into your prayer time. Re-live this passage from Genesis every time you pray.

Allow yourself to relax in the Lord and to breathe deeply from your abdomen and your diaphragm as you pray. Thus your prayer will be not only a prayer of words but also a prayer of gratitude for the gift of life with which you have been blessed.

Gracious Father, thank You for the breath of life. Help me to re-learn the proper breathing techniques I had when I was an infant so that all my cells may receive life-giving oxygen. Thank You for filling me every moment with Your holy, healing breath. In Jesus' name, I pray, Amen.

†

DAY 12
MOVE YOUR BODY

Let them praise his name in the dance: let them sing praises unto him with the timbrel and harp. (Psalm 149:3)

Man goeth forth unto his work and to his labour until the evening. (Psalm 104:23)

Human beings were not created to sit still all day long behind desks or the wheel of an automobile. Our bodies were made to walk, run, bend, turn, and stretch. Unfortunately for the large majority of adults and children in this country, we now have to schedule periods of exercise into our sedentary lives in order to maintain good health.

Movement was meant to be such an integral part of our lives that the concept of "exercise" would be puzzling. Paul, who said in 1 Timothy 4:8 that "bodily exercise profiteth little," was the same guy who routinely walked miles in a single day. He was simply contrasting the benefits of godliness to physical exercise and emphasizing the importance of the Word of God and prayer.

Every system of the body needs movement in order to function normally. Circulation of the blood accelerates, breathing increases, lymphatic fluid moves, the glands and organs are stimulated and massaged. Toxins are flushed from our tissues, fat is burned instead of stored, and cells bustle with life and activity. The bowels work regularly, muscles are toned, and weight is normalized. Movement affects not only our physical self but also our emotional self. Many people who are depressed find that their spirits are lifted and normalized simply by taking regular walks. Endorphins flow and soon they are humming as they walk along.

If you feel ill, do not stop moving your body. If you are currently unable to walk, then move whatever body parts that you can. Begin slowly, increasing activity each day. "No pain, no gain" is a foolhardy philosophy.

Movement should be pleasurable, and you can increase your stamina by extending yourself without reaching a point of pain. If you are not smiling and praising God while you are exercising, consider doing something else! Some people like to skate; some like to play tennis; some like to walk briskly.

Whatever you do, offer your exercise to the Lord and rejoice!

Dear Heavenly Father, I have been sedentary for too long. I praise Your name by moving my body and using it according to your purpose and design. Through movement and work, I stimulate all the systems of my body to function better, and I glorify Your name through my exercise. In Jesus' name, I pray, Amen.

✝

Day 13
Find The Work
God Wants You To Do

Commit thy works unto the Lord, and thy thoughts shall be established. (Proverbs 16:3)

Commit your life's work to God and enjoy it. Find your passion. Some people seem to be born knowing the work that they want to do. At an early age they begin walking a path that they feel guided toward. Others of us flounder around, going from one thing to another, often plodding along in jobs we do not like. For one reason or another, we allow ourselves to get trapped into occupations that do not stimulate or revitalize us.

Whatever your current situation is, stop right this moment and check in with God about His mission for you. Ask Him if you are doing what He would have you to do. Then listen for the answer. If the answer doesn't come today, keep asking until you receive your reply. When you are doing what God wants you to do, you will feel excited, energized by your work, and motivated by a sense of purpose.

How does having meaningful work relate to your health? Those who are unhappy in their work often fall prey to illness. If you are not spending your day engaged in activity that is God's plan for you, then you are not walking in

God's will, and you will probably be subjected to many internal stresses. You may feel frustrated or overwhelmed, bored or fatigued, restless or unfulfilled. These negative emotions take a toll on your physical health. Illness often provides a way out – or at least a break from the job that is literally killing you.

No matter what your past, you always have the present moment. Do not play victim to your work. Take responsibility for your part in following God's plan for your life. If you are unhappy, ask God for direction and guidance. Find out if you are in the right field and if you are living in God's plan, purpose, and design for you. Banish any fears that may try to attack you. Do not let thoughts of "I'm too old to go back to school" or "How will I support myself?" stop you from getting on God's path for you. It is never too late to get in harmony with God's plan for your life.

When your heart is in agreement with God, then your mind, body, and emotions follow.

Dear God, today I will take some time to check in with You about my life's work. Am I doing today what You want me to do? Is this the way I can serve You best? I want to live with zest and enthusiasm, acting as a powerful witness to Your glory. I await quietly Your instruction. In the blessed name of Your Son, Jesus Christ, my Savior and my Redeemer, I pray, Amen.

Focus on leadership. you lead some now. Soon you will lead many. Lead by example.

✝

DAY 14
STRESS CAN KILL YOU

Come unto me, all ye that labour and are heavy laden, and I will give you rest. Take my yoke upon you, and learn of me; for I am meek and lowly in heart: and ye shall find rest unto your souls. For my yoke is easy, and my burden is light. (Matthew 11:28-30)

Stress kills. One of the most difficult lessons for many people is to learn to rest in the Lord. We proclaim faith with our lips and yet worry ourselves into stress, illness, and sometimes even death. We profess the Lord as our Savior and yet live frantic lives, racing from one "to-do" list to the next, never stepping back to ask the Lord to guide our path and set our priorities.

Jesus knows very well that high stress levels make people sick, and, if relief is not found, those illnesses often become fatal ones. Negative stress causes physiological changes throughout the body and especially taxes the nervous system. It also causes constriction of blood vessels, threatening the health of the heart, brain, eyes, organs, and glands.

"Handling" stress is really not the solution. You need a method of living that neutralizes and transforms what the world calls stressful. It is Jesus Christ who can perform the transformation for you. He tells you clearly that He will exchange all the burdens you have for His own yoke, which He says is light and easy.

Jesus does not say you will have no yoke at all, but what He does promise is that He will take the one that is overwhelming to you and will give you one instead that is light enough for you to carry easily.

Are you feeling overwhelmed by the situations in your life? Do you have health problems? Or financial problems? Or relationship problems? Or career problems? Or all of them? Is there too much to do and too little time? Do you dare to trust that Jesus means what He says when He tells you to give your problems to Him?

First, get clear about what your stress is really about. Write down all the things that are having a negative impact on you at the present time. Now, sit in a comfortable chair, close your eyes, quieten your mind, hold your list in your hand, and offer it to Christ Jesus. Ask for guidance in your life and then be bold to follow it.

Heavenly Father, I sometimes feel stress try to overtake me. Jesus told me to give Him my burdens, so I offer them up now. I gladly take His yoke and rest confidently in the knowledge that it is easy and light. Thank You, Father, for showing me the way through Jesus and for restoring peace to my soul. Thank You for lifting me up. Keep teaching me, Father. In Jesus' name, I pray, Amen.

†

Day 15
Rest Is Essential

He maketh me to lie down in green pastures. (Psalm 23:2)

Rest is essential for healing. In order to be restored, we must lie down and be physically still. When we are up and moving around, our bodies use large amounts of energy just to carry out the activities we are performing. While we are in a state of rest, the cells of our body can go about the task of repair and renewal.

We generally think of using energy to do vigorous activity and discount the effort it takes to perform simple, ordinary acts of living. When you are extremely ill, it is difficult simply to talk. You feel fatigue in every part of your body. Trying to form words with your mouth and to summon the strength to push air from your diaphragm past your vocal cords seems a giant task. An action you did without effort thousands of times a day suddenly takes on new dimensions, and you realize how much energy is actually required to speak one tiny word.

Eating also requires a great deal of energy, so if you are seriously ill, you may find that you do not feel hungry. This is the body's natural response so that it can focus its energy in healing rather than in performing the task of digestion. Adequate nutrition is vital, however, to provide the building blocks for recovery, so you may find that eating soup, vegetable juices, and nourishing broth provides the right balance between reducing the demands of digestion and providing the proper intake of nutrients.

Take time to ask God for guidance about the rest you need. Lie down (without allowing any feelings of guilt) when guidance from the Holy Spirit tells you to do so. Make sure you are hearing the Holy Spirit clearly because the enemy would have you use sleep and rest to retreat from the world.

Rest is not meant to be a hiding place. It is meant to be a healing time in the green pastures of restoration where the Lord, your Shepherd, watches lovingly over you and returns you to health.

Loving Father, there are times when I feel tired and weary. I know that I should stop and take time to rest, but instead I keep on pushing ahead without seeking Your counsel and wisdom. When I forget to listen to Your voice, teach me to lie down and turn to Your Word. Thank You, Father, for being my Shepherd, for guarding me, protecting me, and watching over me as I rest. In these green pastures, I rest in You, Your strength, and Your love. I receive my healing through the precious shed blood of my Lord and Savior, Jesus Christ, in whose name I pray, Amen.

✝

DAY 16
GIVE YOURSELF A MINI-RETREAT

And in the morning, rising up a great while before day, he went out, and departed into a solitary place, and there prayed. (Mark 1:35)

And straightway he constrained his disciples to get into the ship, and to go to the other side before unto Bethsaida, while he sent away the people. And when he had sent them away, he departed into a mountain to pray. (Mark 6:45-46)

Do you allow yourself time alone for spiritual renewal? Do you take the time to get away from your family, your friends, and your responsibilities so that you can pray and talk things over with God?

Scripture often describes Jesus as being constantly besieged by people who streamed after Him and pressed around Him. Most of us are not famous and do not have crowds following us. Nevertheless, we, too, have the pressure of daily duties that sometimes seem to us to be a relentless burden instead of a joyous service to God.

When that happens, we must learn to imitate Jesus, our perfect model, and go to a solitary place. Maybe it means getting in the car and going off for an overnight respite. Or maybe it means sending family away for a day, taking the telephone off the hook, setting aside all the laundry and the cleaning and the yard work – then simply resting, praying, and meditating.

It takes courage to take a time out. You can always think of a thousand reasons why you can't do it right now. Maybe in a week – or a month. The fact is that the father of lies deceives you by making you think you "can't" stop. Everyone needs to stop for revitalization and to reaffirm and restore priorities. Jesus was not sick and yet He needed time alone.

When you feel sick or are involved in any form of physical recovery, you need this time even more. Time alone is critical for rest, renewal, and rejuvenation. Turn your mind off and set your worries aside. Allow your body to relax, and allow your heart to float in God's peace and God's love.

Almighty God, give me the courage to take time to rest and to focus on You. I get tangled in my daily activities, and I push through them even when I feel tired. Help me to find a quiet place where I can hear You speak to me. In the stillness of Your peace, I honor You, worship You, and praise You. I thank You for nurturing me, guiding me, and loving me. In the name of Your Son, Christ Jesus, my Savior and my Redeemer, I pray, Amen.

†

DAY 17
DON'T FORGET TO PLAY

And they brought young children to him, that he should touch them: and his disciples rebuked those that brought them. But when Jesus saw it, he was much displeased, and said unto them, Suffer the little children to come unto me, and forbid them not: for of such is the kingdom of God. Verily I say unto you, Whosoever shall not receive the kingdom of God as a little child, he shall not enter therein. And he took them up in his arms, put his hands upon them, and blessed them. (Mark 10:13-16)

Every born-again believer is a child of God, but we often lose sight of that identity because we take ourselves so seriously as adults. Children, unless they are burdened early in life, have a light-hearted way of looking at their world. They know how to play and how to have fun.

It is time for you to lighten up! Illness can weigh you down with problems, worries, and fatigue. Little by little, every task becomes heavy, and you smile less and less. Your face develops worry lines and the twinkle leaves your eyes. Make the decision to lighten up and brighten up. Cast your cares on the Lord and decide to make a joyful noise to Him instead.

Find some outlet for play in your life. Do you like jokes? Find someone to be your "laugh partner" to share funny stories that tickle your funny bone. Do you like to play

53

sports? Find a team and join it. Do you like board games? Ask a couple of friends to have a weekly game with you. Do you like to swing? "Adopt" a neighbor's child and take him to the park.

When at all possible, have some play activities that you do with adults and other play activities that you do with children. You will respond differently emotionally to children than you do to adults and, therefore, the physiological effects will be slightly different.

The more deep-down belly laughter you experience when you play, the healthier you will become. Your glands release many beneficial substances during happy play, and you will feel your body and your emotions becoming lighter and brighter.

Psalm 100:1 says to "make a joyful noise unto the Lord." Father God is delighted when His children rejoice, and He loves the sound of laughter. Be glad and praise the Lord with some play today!

Dear Heavenly Father, You are my all-loving parent who never fails me or lets me down. Teach me to come to you as a little child. Teach me to play at Your feet in the safety and security of Your love. I choose to let joy and laughter fill my body and my soul. I choose to make a joyful noise to You, Father, and to enjoy the healing power of play. In the name of Your Son, Jesus Christ, my Savior and my Redeemer, I pray, Amen.

✝

DAY 18
FIND CREATIVE PLAY OUTLETS

Then were there brought unto him little children, that he should put his hands on them, and pray: and the disciples rebuked them. But Jesus said, Suffer [allow the] little children, and forbid them not, to come unto me: for of such is the kingdom of heaven. And he laid his hands on them, and departed thence.
(Matthew 19:13-15)

Jesus valued children. He liked to have them around and scolded His disciples from keeping the little ones away from Him. Children teach us many important lessons. One that is especially vital to our health is to appreciate play. Good old-fashioned fun.

Play involves laughter, joy, and delight, but it is more than that. Play stimulates our creative qualities and encourages us to expand our heart.

If you feel sick, it is vital that you bring play into your life. One of the best and most obvious ways to do that is to be around the play experts – young children, of course. If you do not have young children of your own and are able, "adopt" a child for a "play day" occasionally. Whether it is for an hour or two, an afternoon, or an entire day, spend time with children – playing games, reading, walking in the park, talking. Being with them will fill your heart with joy and will awaken you to the simple delights of a very young soul.

Not only will you be helping yourself, but you will be a godsend to grateful parents who can have a little time to meet their own needs. There are children everywhere who will bloom with your attention and love.

If you do not feel well enough to supervise a young one, go to a park and watch the children there. Smile and laugh along with them. Join them in your mind if you are not able to join them with your body. (Sadly, there are people who watch children these days with evil intent, so use wisdom when in public places where children are gathered.)

Another way to make contact is by being a pen pal to a child. You can write short notes and stories and send little trinkets from time to time, such as a new barrette or a toy car. In return, your child can draw pictures for you or share a flower or a pebble he found just for you.

Be creative in thinking up a way to bring the play of children into your life. There is much healing in a child's smile, and there are many lessons to learn from seeing a small hand reach for yours.

Father God, help me to discover the child inside myself who likes to play. Help me to look at the world with the delight of young eyes and to sparkle with joy. There is much healing in laughter. Bring me a child who loves jokes, Father, and who can teach me to lighten up, laugh, and rejoice. In the name of Your Son, Jesus Christ, I pray, Amen.

Section Two

Good Nutrition
For
Healthy Living

God's Word has many tips for good nutrition.
Sometimes wisdom is tucked away
in just one word or one brief mention
of a food or herb.
Let's take a look at a few of these nutrition tips
from the Lord.

✝

DAY 19
THE LORD BLESSES OUR FOOD

And ye shall serve the Lord your God, and he shall bless thy bread, and thy water; and I will take sickness away from the midst of thee.   (Exodus 23:25)

For it is sanctified by the word of God and prayer.
(1 Timothy 4:5)

The Scripture in Exodus exhorts us to serve the Lord. We are to let every breath and every action be joyful worship of our God, who is the Great I AM. Worshipping God means going to Him with honor and with reverence and giving Him an exalted place in your heart and in your life. When you do this, what does this Scripture say will happen?

This passage gives us a bit of a surprise for an answer. It tells us that God's blessing will be on your food and water. That certainly seems to take us from the sublime to the mundane, doesn't it? Let's see now, when you serve and honor God, He will bless your food and water.

We find a connection between the Old Covenant passage in Exodus and the New Covenant passage in 1 Timothy 4:5. "For it [our food] is sanctified by the word of God and prayer." Food and water provide the basic nutrition that we need in order for our bodies to be healthy. Since God wants us to be healthy, He needs for us to eat the proper foods that will nourish and sustain us. When we sit down to eat, God wants to bless our food. He wants to keep us healthy and strong.

We are given the responsibility to make wise food choices to provide the best nutrients for our body that we can. When we do our part, we can count on the blessings of our Heavenly Father.

As Christians, when we sit down to eat, we "say a blessing" over our food and water. We do it partly to remind ourselves of God's sovereignty and grace in our lives. But we also do it because God's blessing on our food and water is integral to our physical vitality.

At your next meal, bow your head and thank God for blessing your food and water. Don't speak the words mechanically, but instead pray with conviction and purpose. Eat slowly and know that you are receiving not only nutritious food for your body but also the power and healing love of God.

Father God, thank You for the abundance of the foods that You have provided for me. I do my best to eat pure, wholesome, organic food as You designed it because I understand the importance of unadulterated food for the health of my body. I ask Your guidance in selecting the foods that You want me to eat. I worship You as my God and my Creator. Thank You for always blessing my food and my water so that I may be strong in fulfilling Your purpose for my life. In Jesus' name, I pray, Amen.

†

Day 20
What Foods Are Best To Eat?

My son, eat thou honey, because it is good; and the honeycomb, which is sweet to thy taste: So shall the knowledge of wisdom be unto thy soul: when thou hast found it, then there shall be a reward, and thy expectation shall not be cut off.
(Proverbs 24:13-14)

This Proverb compares the sweetness of the taste of honey to the sweetness of the "knowledge of wisdom" for your soul. When you have found this knowledge of wisdom, there is a future for you.

God's health laws are among the wisdom we have to be willing to seek. If we find them, there is a future for us, and our lives will not be cut off prematurely by our own foolishness and disobedience.

How do we know what foods are wise choices and which are unwise? Turn to God's Holy Scripture. First, look for things that God specifically tells us are to be food for us. Read Genesis 1:29 (seeds, nuts, fruits, and vegetables) and Genesis 3:18 (plants of the field), for example. Also read Leviticus 11:2-23 (animals that are not scavengers because scavengers consume toxins and carry many parasites, bacteria, and viruses).

Second, look for items that God tells us not to eat. Read Leviticus 7:23 (cover fat of cattle, sheep, or goats) and

Deuteronomy 12:16 (blood of animals). But don't get into a legalistic box regarding food. Remember the admonition in 1 Timothy 4:4, "For every creature of God is good and nothing to be refused, if it be received with thanksgiving."

Third, look for edible things that God gives as gifts. Read Ezekiel 16:19 (whole grain flour, olive oil, and honey) and Exodus 16:13-15 (quail).

Fourth, look for food that Jesus ate or gave to others to eat. Read Matthew 15:36 (whole grain bread and fish) and Isaiah 7:15 (curds and honey).

Fifth, look for food that Jesus used in His stories and parables. Read Matthew 7:9-11 (fish and whole grain bread) and Luke 11:11-13 (fish and eggs).

God blessed our bodies with thousands of internal healing mechanisms. In order for them to function properly, we have to provide our bodies with appropriate food and nutrition. We must seek the wisdom that will provide us with a healthy future according to God's plan.

Almighty God, sometimes I want my future the easy way – my way. I seek Your wisdom and instruction about Your health guidelines. Only in Your wisdom is there a future for me. Teach me, Father. In the precious name of Jesus, I pray, Amen.

✝

DAY 21
ARE SOME FOODS "UNCLEAN?"

... These are the beasts which ye shall eat among all the beasts that are on the earth. Whatsoever parteth the hoof, and is clovenfooted, and cheweth the cud, among the beasts, that shall ye eat. ... These shall ye eat of all that are in the waters: whatsoever hath fins and scales in the waters, in the seas, and in the rivers, them shall ye eat. (Leviticus 11:2-3, 9)

Now the spirit speaketh expressly, that in the latter times some shall depart from the faith, giving heed to seducing spirits, and doctrines of devils; ... commanding to abstain from meats, which God created to be received with thanksgiving of them which believe and know the truth. For every creature of God is good, and nothing to be refused, if it be received with thanksgiving: for it is sanctified by the word of God and prayer. (1 Timothy 4:1, 3-5)

There are some Christians who believe that the Old Testament rules of clean and unclean foods apply to them, although the majority of Christians follow the Scripture written by Paul to Timothy where he states that it is a "doctrine of devils" to forbid someone to abstain from meats. Is there a way to reconcile these two views?

As Christians, we clearly have been delivered from the curse of the law and are not bound to the requirements of Mosaic law. But before we dismiss Leviticus as antiquated and out-of-date, let's take a closer look at the animals named there.

The animals that are classified as "unclean" have a common characteristic – they are able to sustain a high level of bacteria, viruses, and parasites without themselves dying. Many of them are scavengers because God needed a clean-up crew of animals that would eat toxic material and garbage and still be able to survive.

In 1953 a study was done at Johns Hopkins University by Dr. David Macht to record the toxins found in the flesh of various animals. Here is what is so fascinating. His results showed that the animals, birds, and fish with the highest levels of toxins in their flesh matched the list of unclean animals given in Leviticus 11. Likewise, the animals with the lowest levels of toxins in their flesh matched the list of clean animals given in Leviticus 11. That is certainly worth noting. Let me repeat his findings. The animals that were declared "unclean" in Leviticus had the highest levels of toxins in their flesh.

What should we do? Can we eat any food that we want to eat? As Christians redeemed by the blood of Jesus, the answer is absolutely yes. But Paul said that even though anything was allowable for him, not everything was the wisest for him.

For myself, most of the time I choose to eat foods that I believe have the least amounts of toxins. I consider the food list in Leviticus to be a warning to me of potential problems with high toxic levels of foods; therefore, I generally choose to eat the foods in the "clean" category. In today's world there are many other issues that relate to the safety and quality of food, such as the saturation of different foods with pesticides and the exposure of foods to E. coli and other harmful organisms. For example, I do not eat conventionally grown apples because they are so heavily sprayed. Instead, I choose apples that are organically grown.

God has always wanted us to be healthy, and He filled His Word with guidance about proper nutrition. As you walk on your path to your healing, pay attention to the foods you eat and let the Holy Spirit lead you to make healthy choices.

Blessed Creator, thank You for providing guidelines in Your Holy Word to tell me which foods are healthiest for me to eat. I will do my part in providing my body the best nutrition I can. In Jesus' name, I pray, Amen.

✝

DAY 22
MORE ON CLEAN AND UNCLEAN FOODS

Then came together unto him the Pharisees, and certain of the scribes, which came from Jerusalem. And when they saw some of his disciples eat bread with defiled, that is to say, with unwashen, hands, they found fault. For the Pharisees, and all the Jews, except they wash their hands oft, eat not, holding the tradition of the elders. (Mark 7:1-3)

And he ... said unto them, Hear, and understand: Not that which goeth into the mouth defileth a man; but that which cometh out of the mouth, this defileth a man. ... But those things which proceed out of the mouth come forth from the heart; and they defile the man. For out of the heart proceed evil thoughts, murders, adulteries, fornications, thefts, false witness, blasphemies: these are the things which defile a man: but to eat with unwashen hands defileth not a man. (Matthew 15:10-11, 18-20)

We continue our exploration of the issue of clean and unclean foods as we look at the way that Jesus confronted traditions of men. According to Jewish law, people became spiritually unclean when they ate foods God had declared to be unclean. Likewise, they became defiled if they ate without washing their hands first.

In His reply to the scribes and Pharisees, Jesus made it clear that the state of a person's heart has nothing to do with what foods they do or do not eat. Nor, He says, does eating with unwashed hands make a person unclean spiritually.

Was Jesus saying that it is best to eat with dirty hands? Of course not. Jesus was not addressing a health or sanitation issue. He was addressing a moral and spiritual issue.

Just as it is not healthy to eat with unwashed hands because the risk of contaminating our food is high, it is also not healthy to eat animals which carry an especially high level of toxins because the risk of contaminating our body with bacteria, viruses, and parasites is high. It is well known that a large proportion of food poisoning in humans comes after we eat pork or shellfish.

God wants us to be well. Learn what food recommendations were given to us. Then ask God how best to apply what you have learned to your life.

Loving Father, in studying Your Word, I am learning about the foods that You have told me are less healthy to eat than others. I know that all food that I bless in the name of Jesus is safe for me. Help me to choose the most wholesome foods to eat as I become a full partner with You in my healing process. In Jesus' name, I pray, Amen.

†

DAY 23
HOW DO YOU CHANGE
YOUR EATING HABITS?

When thou sittest to eat with a ruler, consider diligently what is before thee: and put a knife to thy throat, if thou be a man given to appetite. Be not desirous of his dainties: for they are deceitful meat. (Proverbs 23:1-3)

People have not changed much since the days when Proverbs was written. Look at some of the primary health problems in our country – obesity, diabetes, heart attacks, cancer, peptic ulcer, hiatal hernia, hemorrhoids, varicose veins, appendicitis, and gallstones, just to name a few. There is a nutritional component to each of these ailments, and we must take responsibility for the willful choices we are making in our diets. Too much processed salt, too much refined sugar, too few vegetables, too little pure water, too little fiber. To make poor choices and then to blame God for the result by calling our illness His will is unfair, to say the least.

Most of us do not know how to make the shift from unhealthy foods to healthy ones. We have in our mind that we will have to eat food that looks like grass and tastes like hay, and we decide that we would rather be dead than eat that! Unfortunately, many people end up sacrificing their lives because they believe that lie of the evil one.

Begin gradually and take one step at a time. Start by drinking pure water, one-half ounce for each pound of body weight. Add one lightly steamed vegetable to your diet every three days until you are eating at least four (preferably more) vegetables a day. Make the extra effort to get organic produce as often as possible because, when you feel sick, you need to remove the toxic load from your liver.

To keep the same food amounts on your plate as you add more vegetables, simply reduce the portion sizes of the other items. Now add a little fresh fruit to your diet in the same gradual manner. Use it for a snack instead of soft drinks, cookies, and candy bars. Next, reduce the meat that you are eating to only once per day. Shift to hormone-free and antibiotic-free chicken, turkey, and fish. Add more beans to your diet.

Now that I've given you some suggestions, let me tell you not to follow them until you seek confirmation and direction from the Holy Spirit. People often get into trouble because they follow this diet or that diet or this health expert or that herbalist because they make assumptions that whatever they are told is the "right" thing to do. The rules may be "right" for 99 percent of the people on the planet - but maybe, just maybe, the Holy Spirit knows a reason why it is not best for you at this precise moment.

So be sure you ask for guidance whether these - or any other - nutrition guidelines are appropriate and healthy for you to follow. Let the Holy Spirit be your daily guide. Then, as you make the changes in your diet that the Holy Spirit tells you to make and you begin to feel the difference in your body and health, give grateful thanks to God for healing you.

Almighty God, I really like certain foods that I know are not healthy for me. I need Your help in making a commitment to follow Your will for my diet instead of helping the enemy destroy my health. Help me to make the changes You would have me to make. Show me exactly what You want me to do, and I will do it. In Jesus' name, I pray, Amen.

✝

DAY 24
SHOULD YOU FAST?

Moreover when ye fast, be not, as the hypocrites, of a sad countenance: for they disfigure their faces, that they may appear unto men to fast. Verily I say unto you, They have their reward. But thou, when thou fastest, anoint thine head, and wash thy face; that thou appear not unto men to fast, but unto thy Father which is in secret: and thy Father, which seeth in secret, shall reward thee openly. (Matthew 6:16-18)

Fasting was a common spiritual practice in the time of Jesus, but few people fast today, either for spiritual or health reasons. From a health standpoint, when you fast, you make a determination to refrain from eating either all foods or certain foods for a certain period of time. This slows digestion so the energy of the body can be shifted to repairing organs and cells which need healing.

The purpose of spiritual fasting is to force your body to accept the fact that spiritual reality is superior to physical reality. During the period of fasting, you spend the maximum amount of time reading the Bible and communicating with God through prayer. You enforce on your body the truth that you "esteem the words of his mouth more than (your) necessary food" (Job 23:12).

As you focus on worship, you train your body to obey spiritual truth rather than to obey the physical demands of hunger pangs. In a very powerful and significant way, this helps you to learn to see beyond your symptoms to God's truth of healing.

Even though it is generally healthy to fast, do not assume that fasting is a wise choice for you. Ask the Holy Spirit first. Ask if you are to undertake a fast, and, if so, what kind and how long.

If your body is very weak and you go on a three-day water fast without asking for guidance first, you may delay your recovery instead of accelerating it. Or if your pancreas is malfunctioning and you go on a three-day fruit fast without asking for guidance, you can create serious imbalances with your blood sugar levels. If you had asked for guidance, you might have been told to go on a vegetable fast for two days.

Always ask for guidance first whenever you have a decision to make regarding your health and recovery.

Father God, I esteem Your Words more than my necessary food. I want to strengthen my spiritual muscles and am considering a fast. Reveal to me through the Holy Spirit if I should begin a fast, and, if so, tell me exactly what kind of fast to do and what its length should be. I will be obedient to the guidance that I receive. In the name of Your Son, Jesus Christ, Amen.

✝

DAY 25
THE VALUE OF HERBS

... the earth is satisfied with the fruit of thy works. He causeth the grass to grow for the cattle, and the herb for the service of man: that he may bring forth food out of the earth. (Psalm 104:13-14)

The Psalms were written to expound the glory of the Lord God Almighty, and in the process, many health truths are shared with us. This Psalm reveals to us one of the fundamental laws of nutrition: that the source of nutrients for us is found in the plants.

What do plants need in order to live? Minerals, water, air, and sunlight. The plants take in these elements and process them. Their leaves, flowers, stems, and roots then become loaded with a myriad of substances necessary for our nutrition and for our healing.

Herbs are plants that have dense amounts of healing nutrients, and essential oils are the lifeblood of the plants. Consequently, they are applied and consumed in much smaller quantities than "ordinary" foods. For example, we usually eat smaller servings of garlic than we do of string beans, and we apply tiny amounts of dill essential oil compared to the amount we would use as a seasoning.

What most people do not know is that plants are our best source of minerals. God created the plants to be able to take the minerals from the soil and package them in a way in which the human body can digest and assimilate them. We can eat the rock and the soil directly (which is the source of many mineral supplements today); however, when we consume them in that form, we assimilate very little of it. Our bodies were not designed to digest rock.

Most of us eat meat and fish, and Scripture provides guidelines for us to do so in the healthiest way. However, if we rely on animal products as the major component of our diet, we are depending on second-hand food for our own nutrition.

God intended that we get a large portion of our nutrition firsthand from plants. The plants, herbs, and essential oils are truly "for the service of man."

Almighty God, You created this glorious world in which I live. I have taken much of it for granted and have too often failed to give proper value to the plants which You provided in such abundance. As I learn more about the way that my body works, I appreciate the function of plants in filling my body's needs for nutrients. I choose to eat appropriate amounts of fruits and vegetables for my health. How grateful I am for the herbs and essential oils which You gave for my service. In Jesus' name, I pray, Amen.

†

Day 26
Our Bodies Love Herbs

... and the fruit thereof shall be for meat [food], and the leaf thereof for medicine [healing]. (Ezekiel 47:12)

Have you ever thought about the staggering abundance of herbs that exist on our beautiful planet Earth? Do you believe they are the result of an accidental process or do you believe that each plant was created with specific intent for a specific purpose by a Loving Creator?

As part of God's creation, herbs are vibrantly alive and each one has been created by our loving Father, who spoke it into existence by His Word. Every herb has a unique purpose in our world.

It is interesting that each part of creation instinctively recognizes another part of creation. Each cell of our body has its own intelligence implanted by the Lord God Almighty and operates according to that divine plan without our having to tell it to do so. This cellular knowing enables it to respond to God's herbal creations differently than it does with man's creations, which do not have God's breath of life.

For example, the body recognizes and processes beneficial herbs as concentrated foods and puts them to immediate use. On the other hand, the body identifies pharmaceutical drugs as something foreign to the body and not found in nature and thus generally tries to filter them from the body by various mechanisms. Dosages are calculated to override this process so that the drug can perform its intended function.

God's herbs (and the essential oils within these herbs) are intended to be used to restore balance to our bodies. Learn about these precious treasures given by your loving, compassionate Heavenly Father.

Before taking them, seek guidance from the Holy Spirit so that you will use them wisely for the purpose they were intended. Then say "Thank You" to your Heavenly Father.

O, wonderful Creator, I bow in awe to You, to Your glory and majesty. Thank You for the plants which You declared to me to be for food, and thank You for herbs and essential oils which You provided for my health and healing. Lead me, Father, to a greater understanding of how Your herbs work according to Your plan for my healing. Give me the perseverance to learn all I can about them, and give me the guidance to use them for my best and highest good. In Jesus' name, I pray, Amen.

✝

DAY 27
THE DIET FOR A PERFECT WORLD

And God said, Behold, I have given you every herb bearing seed, which is upon the face of all the earth, and every tree, in the which is the fruit of a tree yielding seed; to you it shall be for meat [food]. (Genesis 1:29)

In the first chapter of Genesis, God creates us, His beloved children, and now He needs to get us started on the right track. He has two initial things to say. The first is that we are to have dominion over the earth. The second instruction is largely overlooked and ignored. The bottom line is: eat plants for food.

What? Yes, that means fruits and vegetables. The essential nature of plants is for our nutrition and wellness, and we cannot be healthy without them because God ordained this from the first moment of our creation.

Am I advocating that we eat the "Genesis" diet as our only source of food? No, for several reasons. First, this was a diet for a perfect world. The plants yielding the food grew easily, and Adam simply picked it and ate it. We no longer live in a perfect world. The ground is now cursed, and it yields only after we toil to farm it. Disease now exists, both for us and for the plants. The changes were profound and catastrophic.

Second, God gave specific new instructions for us to eat animal products. In Genesis 9:3, God said to Noah after the flood, "I have given them [animals] to you for food, just as I have given you grain and vegetables. But you must never eat any meat that still has the lifeblood in it" (New Living Translation). Then more instructions were given in Leviticus.

If someone chooses to eat according to the original instructions in Genesis 1:29 and he recovers from illness, that is wonderful. Everyone is free to follow what the Holy Spirit leads him to do. However, I do not think it is scripturally sound to say that the diet given in Genesis is the "best" or only correct diet to follow.

What God is making clear in Genesis is that vegetables, fruit, and nuts are part of good nutrition for us. Unfortunately, many people today "don't like" vegetables and consider their French-fried potatoes and a little iceberg lettuce in a hamburger to be their vegetables for the day. Our government once even declared ketchup to be a vegetable. Children are often allowed to fill up on snacks loaded with sugar, and, consequently, they aren't hungry at mealtime for nutritious food.

Even more sadly, we have allowed our lives to become so hectic and frantically filled with activities that we don't have time to prepare healthy meals. The more stressed we are, the less time we take to prepare what we know is nutritious for our bodies.

Take a look at your own meals. Food was so important that God told you from the very beginning what to eat. How many fruits and vegetables do you include in your daily diet? Are some of them eaten raw? Plants are filled with enzymes to aid in digestion but heat destroys some of these substances. How many of your vegetables are overcooked, saturated with pesticides, and covered with margarine and processed salt?

What you eat has a major role in the state of your health because your cells depend on the nutrients you give them. How ridiculous to disregard God's instructions willfully and then blame Him when your body breaks down and you feel ill.

Take responsibility for your health. Ask forgiveness for abusing your body, and then eat the right foods to support its healing.

Almighty Creator, thank You for this marvelous earth. You have given me a vast array of plants to eat for food and a multitude of herbs, not only to use for food but also to help my body heal when it is sick. I seek to learn more about Your plants and herbs so that I will be a good steward over all these many gifts. With grateful thanks, in Jesus' name, I pray, Amen.

✝

DAY 28
SHOULD YOU BE A VEGETARIAN?

One man's faith allows him to eat everything, but another man, whose faith is weak, eats only vegetables. The man who eats everything must not look down on him who does not, and the man who does not eat everything must not condemn the man who does, for God has accepted him. ...

He who eats meat, eats to the Lord, for he gives thanks to God; and he who abstains, does so to the Lord and gives thanks to God. (Romans 14:2-3, 6   New International Version)

A great deal of debate rages both in the natural health arena and in various religious denominations whether it is "best" to be a vegetarian. Many theories have been offered and it would be impossible to follow them all.

Some people say we should eat the diet described in Genesis 1. The instruction in the perfect, sinless world of the Garden of Eden was for Adam and Eve to eat fruits, vegetables, seeds, and nuts. Later after the fall, meat was introduced and specific instructions were given in Genesis, Exodus, and Leviticus.

Daniel ate a vegetarian diet when taken into the palace of the king; however, it is reasonable to assume that he ate a traditional Jewish diet (which included lamb and other meat) both prior to his captivity and after he was no longer enslaved.

We know from the Word that Jesus ate fish and prepared it for His disciples. As we examine the Scripture, there is nothing that indicates that Jesus had a diet different from the normal foods of the Jewish culture, such as lamb, eggs, bread, and milk.

Here in Romans, Paul describes a vegetarian as a person whose faith is weaker than a person who eats meat, but he plainly states that neither the vegetarians nor the meat-eaters should condemn each other. Simply eat whatever you eat to the glory of God.

What are you supposed to do? Study the Word to see what God tells you about healthy foods. Be open to hearing the opinions of natural health and medical professionals, yet do not feel compelled to follow any of them.

Sometimes following the example of Daniel by eating only vegetables and fruits for several days helps a sick person to recover. Do not assume that you should do so, however, without first going to God in prayer and asking what path you should follow.

God created your body, and God knows exactly how it is functioning and what type of nutrients it needs. Ask the Holy Spirit to reveal to you what you should eat, including specifics such as frequency, method of cooking, etc. He will show you the proper nutrition for your body.

Father God, I know that what I eat is a major factor in creating the health I seek. I want to eat nutritious foods, and I ask for Your guidance about the exact foods that You want me to eat. I am willing to do as You instruct. Help me to exercise the self-discipline I need to make the changes You ask of me. In Jesus' name, I pray, Amen.

†

DAY 29
THE BENEFITS OF ESSENTIAL OILS

Then took Mary a pound of ointment of spikenard, very costly, and anointed the feet of Jesus, and wiped his feet with her hair: and the house was filled with the odour of the ointment.

Then saith one of his disciples, Judas Iscariot, Simon's son, which should betray him, why was not this ointment sold for three hundred pence, and given to the poor?

This he said, not that he cared for the poor; but because he was a thief, and had the bag, and bare what was put therein.
(John 12:3-6)

Here is a passage of Holy Scripture that connects Jesus with essential oils and points us to God's divine blessing on the use of these oils for healing purposes. Mary anointed Jesus' feet with a pound of very costly ointment, which the King James translation calls spikenard, but which might have been myrrh. Whatever the oil was, we know that it was enormously expensive – so expensive that Judas got very upset because he felt Mary had wasted the oil. He had apparently planned to sell it and take the money for himself.

This Scripture in John says that "the house was filled with the odour of the ointment." This illustrates the aromatic strength of essential oils. Today we often use a device called a diffuser to disperse essential oils throughout one or more rooms in our house. When we inhale the vapor, it goes to our lungs, brain, and blood in seconds and then is carried to all the cells in our body. Different oils have different healing benefits, so selecting the appropriate oil and diffusing it can greatly accelerate your healing process.

Because they are carried swiftly to organs, tissues, and cells in our body, care must be taken to use oils of only the very highest therapeutic grade quality. In addition to being inhaled, essential oils can also be applied to the skin and even in certain cases taken internally as a nutritional supplement. Not all of these methods are appropriate for every oil, so it is important to take some time to learn about essential oils and their proper use.

There are also special techniques to apply particular oils to the entire spinal column, killing viruses and bacteria that hide there. Massaging the oils into the feet is another method of application that is very therapeutic.

There are hundreds of essential oils, and their healing properties are extensive. For example, juniper has been used for centuries for urinary tract infections and for kidney and bladder problems. Birch has been used to strengthen bones and relieve bone and muscle pain. Cedarwood has been used for its purifying action on problems such as acne and skin diseases. Spruce has been used to restore the glandular system, including the pineal, thymus, and adrenal glands. Fir has been used for bronchial problems and respiratory complaints.

Essential oils have many regenerating, detoxifying, and oxygenating qualities. Their molecules pass through cell walls quickly, and some can even penetrate the blood brain barrier which may make them useful to people with brain disorders such as Alzheimer's and Parkinson's disease. Essential oils act to vitalize us and thus help to restore health to us.

How marvelous it is for us to be able to experience the restorative, healing properties of these precious oils that God has given us. Learn about the therapeutic value of essential oils and ask the Holy Spirit if they would be useful for your healing.

Heavenly Father, the aroma of precious essential oils filled the room where Jesus was. I want to learn about essential oils and the way that I can use them to restore health to my body. Send me teachers, Father, and I will learn. You have provided so many healing remedies to me in nature, Father. Help me to use them wisely. In the name of Jesus Christ, my Savior and my Redeemer, I pray, Amen.

†

DAY 30
ANOINTING WITH OIL FOR HEALING

Is any among you afflicted? let him pray. Is any merry? let him sing psalms. Is any sick among you? let him call for the elders of the church; and let them pray over him, anointing him with oil in the name of the Lord:

And the prayer of faith shall save the sick, and the Lord shall raise him up; and if he have committed sins, they shall be forgiven him.

Confess your faults one to another, and pray one for another, that ye may be healed. The effectual fervent prayer of a righteous man availeth much. (James 5:13-16)

James speaks of a specific ordinance for healing consisting of anointing the sick with oil. We are told to call the elders of the church to pray over us and to anoint us with oil in the name of the Lord. The power of this anointing is particularly strong because we are in the midst of those who not only believe in Jesus Christ but who also believe in God's will and ability to heal us. We are anointed by believers who are strong in their faith and whose prayers are not weakened by doubt.

There are few churches today that observe this anointing ordinance. Those that do usually use olive oil or something similar. It is more likely that the disciples and the followers of the early church were taught to use true essential oils which were often diluted in olive oil.

91

In Mark 6 we are told that Jesus sent his disciples out two by two, giving them specific instructions. Verse 13 says that the twelve men returned, reporting that they had "anointed with oil many that were sick and healed them." The Greek word used in this text refers to olive oil because this was the carrier oil that was used to dilute the strongly potent essential oils. "Cutting" the essential oils with olive oil also served the purpose of making a small quantity of essential oils available to a much larger number of people.

We get a clue that the oil had a purpose in more gradual healings by noting that the word "healed" in verse 13 is the Greek word "*therapeuo,*" the basis for the English word "therapy." It means "to relieve of disease" and "to wait upon menially" (i.e. to serve). It is not a word that implies a miraculous, instantaneous healing but rather implies a healing accomplished over a period of time.

We see here that Jesus gave His disciples a universally available and acceptable tool that they could use after He had returned to the Father. God's best is certainly that we receive our healing quickly. But God wants most of all that we get well, and He is always willing to meet us where we are.

Can you follow the instructions of James and anoint with "plain" olive oil? Of course. That is the way it is regularly done where it is practiced today. But it is important to remember what essential oils have potent therapeutic, healing qualities to aid in recovery, and it is instructive to us to think that Jesus probably used them.

Anointing with oil – no matter what kind of oil we use – is done in the name of the Lord. It is done as though Jesus were standing there Himself. And what is the result we can expect? To be healed in our body.

Loving Father, help me to find a church where the faithful will anoint me with oil and pray in Jesus' name for my healing. I need the help of a Christian fellowship that believes in Your healing power and that will encourage me to keep my faith strong. I give grateful thanks to You for Your gracious gift of plants which contain essential oils and which are beneficial to my health and healing. I seek to learn more about them and to use them for the purpose that You have ordained. I am blessed by them and use them in the name of Your Son, Jesus Christ, in whose name I pray, Amen.

†

DAY 31
THE MAGI'S GIFT OF ESSENTIAL OILS TO JESUS

Now when Jesus was born in Bethlehem of Judea, ... behold, there came wise men from the east to Jerusalem, saying, Where is he that is born King of the Jews? for we have seen his star in the east, and are come to worship him. ...

And when they were come into the house, they saw the young child with Mary his mother, and fell down, and worshipped him: and when they had opened their treasures, they presented unto him gifts; gold, and frankincense, and myrrh.   (Matthew 2:1-2, 11)

What gifts would you take to a king? The magi believed they were looking for a child who had been born to be a king, and they wanted to bring Him treasures that reflected their desire to honor and worship Him. Consider their selections. Not one of the three gifts was made by man. No ornate jewelry. No luxurious clothes. No toys.

All three gifts for the Son of God were made by God. They were all items found in nature. Everyone understands gold and recognizes it as a precious metal of great value.

What about frankincense? It is a fragrant gum resin and essential oil that was used for various healing purposes. It was considered to be a holy anointing oil, and its many uses include helping physical problems we now associate with the immune system. It has certain chemical components

95

that stimulate the brain centers for memory and emotions, as well as affecting the hypothalamus gland which produces thyroid and growth hormones.

Like frankincense, myrrh was also a valuable oil, being extremely useful in both oil and herb form for healing due to its strong antiseptic, anti-bacterial, and anti-viral actions. It has been used for such diverse conditions as gum infections, hepatitis, fungal infections, and skin problems.

Just as the wise men expressed their adoration of the newborn king, we, too, worship our Lord and Savior. As we seek to follow His will for us, we, too, can use herbal treasures God gave us in the beginning when He created our universe.

God wants us to be well, so He filled nature with many plants, essential oils, and herbs for our healing. He gave them to us in abundance because He knew our need for them would be great. Our responsibility is to learn about them, to use them wisely according to His purpose and guidance, and to value them as precious gifts from our Heavenly Father.

Most glorious Creator, thank You for the profusion of herbs which You have given to me. You have blessed me with an array of Your healing herbs, essential oils, and natural substances that is so vast that I can hardly comprehend it. Teach me about Your healing remedies, Father. Guide me so that I may learn about them and may use them wisely according to Your will, purpose, and guidance. In Jesus' name, I pray, Amen.

✝

DAY 32
GOD CALLS OLIVE OIL GOOD

Until I come and take you away to a land like your own land, a land of corn and wine, a land of bread and vineyards, a land of oil olive and of honey, that ye may live, and not die. (2 Kings 18:32)

My meat [food] also which I gave thee, fine flour, and oil, and honey, wherewith I fed thee, thou hast even set it before them for a sweet savour: and thus it was, saith the Lord God. (Ezekiel 16:19)

For the Lord thy God bringeth thee into a good land, a land of brooks of water, of fountains and depths that spring out of valleys and hills; a land of wheat, and barley, and vines, and fig trees, and pomegranates; a land of oil olive, and honey; a land wherein thou shalt eat bread without scarceness, thou shalt not lack any thing in it. (Deuteronomy 8:7-9)

The references to olive oil as a good thing and as a gift of God appear over and over again in Holy Scripture. The people in the Mediterranean countries have long used large amounts of olive oil in their cooking, and it is interesting that statistics show that they have low incidences of heart disease.

Since it is a versatile oil, it is useful both as a cooking oil and as a dressing on salads. It contains monounsaturated fats, which we now categorize as a "good" fat because it is used so beneficially in the human body. In addition to its helpful effect in preventing heart disease, it also contains substances such as steric and oleic acid, which may help to prevent breast cancer.

Olive oil may also be used to help in the recovery from particular ailments. Historically, some people have rubbed it nightly over their liver for detoxification. For centuries, people have flushed gallstones from their body by following a specific procedure involving the drinking of a mixture of olive oil and lemon juice.

The Holy Scripture provides a wealth of guidelines for healthy living. When you read God's Word, notice how often references to olive oil as a good thing or a cherished commodity pops up. Consider that this information was supposed to be giving us a clue for helping us to walk in abundant life. So read the Word and learn.

Wonderful Father God, I read Your Word, but often I miss much of Your advice for good nutrition and healthy living. I know that I am responsible for the food that I put into my temple, and I want to do a better job of making wise choices. Today I am taking a new look at olive oil so that I can incorporate it into my diet. Thank You, Father, for the wonderful foods like barley and figs and pomegranates and honey and olive oil that You have provided so that I can walk in perfect health. In the name of Your Son, Jesus Christ, I pray, Amen.

✝

DAY 33
HOW HEZEKIAH WAS HEALED WITH FIGS

Turn again, and tell Hezekiah the captain of my people, Thus saith the Lord, the God of David thy father, I have heard thy prayer, I have seen thy tears: behold, I will heal thee: on the third day thou shalt go up unto the house of the Lord.

And I will add unto thy days fifteen years; and I will deliver thee and this city out of the hand of the king of Assyria; and I will defend this city for mine own sake, and for my servant David's sake.

And Isaiah said, Take a lump of figs. And they took and laid it on the boil, and he recovered. (2 Kings 20:5-7)

Living in the time before Jesus came to atone for all, Hezekiah, king of Judah, is still under the curse of the law. He becomes gravely ill, and the prophet Isaiah goes to him, tells him to prepare for death, and then leaves.

Hezekiah immediately turns to the Lord and cries out to Him. "Remember now how I have walked before thee in truth and with a perfect heart, and have done that which is good in thy sight" (2 Kings 20:3).

God responds to Hezekiah by intercepting Isaiah before he can even get out of the courtyard. "I have heard thy prayer. I have seen thy tears," God says as He extends his mercy to Hezekiah and promises to heal him. In only three days, the healing will be accomplished.

God alone is the Healer, but often natural substances can be used to assist in recovery. In Hezekiah's case, the Lord reveals to Isaiah to prepare a poultice of figs.

We usually think of figs simply as a fruit to eat; however, it is a little-known fact that they are one of the most alkaline of all foods and have a powerful anti-acid effect. Therefore, they have historically been used for ulcers (of both the mouth and the stomach), heartburn, boils on the gums, and also to help remove bad odors from cancers.

Holy Scripture tells us that figs were applied to Hezekiah's boil according to God's instruction, and he recovered.

Let the Holy Spirit show you God's plan for your path to healing. Perhaps, like Hezekiah, it will involve the use of some of His abundant herbs, essential oils, or plants. Be open to whatever guidance you are given and follow it with gratitude.

Father God, thank You that, unlike Hezekiah, I have the sure Word of the New Covenant that Your healing is flowing to me right now. If there are natural remedies that will nourish my body at the physical level, reveal that information to me, and I will follow Your guidance without question or hesitation. Thank You for healing me. In Jesus' name, I pray, Amen.

✝

Day 34
The Healing Benefits Of Garlic

We remember the fish, which we did eat in Egypt freely; the cucumbers, and the melons, and the leeks, and the onions, and the garlic. (Numbers 11:5)

Garlic is a marvelous food which has many powerful health benefits. A member of the onion family, garlic's pungent odor comes from its sulfur compounds, the most commonly known one being allicin.

Used in Biblical times as an antibiotic, garlic is still effective for that purpose today. It is a powerful stimulant to the immune system, and the various natural sulfur compounds that it contains are antagonistic to many types of microorganisms, including flu, colds, viruses, and bacteria. Its anti-viral, anti-bacterial, and anti-fungal actions give it several advantages over many antibiotics.

Throughout the world, garlic has been used to combat intestinal infections, diarrhea, and diseases such as cholera and typhoid. When fighting an infection, people have learned to use small, frequently repeated amounts of either whole cloves of fresh garlic or hi-potency enteric-coated tablets. (Be careful not to select supplements which have had the allicin removed in order to be "odorless.")

Garlic has been used for centuries to lower high blood pressure. It has been shown to improve cholesterol levels by raising HDL cholesterol and lowering LDL cholesterol. It has been used to help with cases of asthma and diabetes.

In addition, it has been used to improve liver and gallbladder function. Garlic helps to remove mucus from the digestive and intestinal tract. It even has anti-cancer properties. Studies are now showing that garlic may even help to improve your personality! People who regularly eat garlic have fewer mood swings and less anxiety, fatigue, and irritability.

Should you eat lots of garlic or take garlic preparations? Just because the list of benefits is long, don't assume that the answer is yes. Go in prayer and ask the Holy Spirit to reveal to you what you should do.

Father God, how grateful I am for the plants which You have provided in great abundance for my health and healing. Show me the best way that I can learn more about them and use them wisely in the way You intended. Teach me, as I seek a closer relationship with You. In the name of Jesus Christ, my Lord and Savior, I pray, Amen.

✝

DAY 35
IS FAT GOOD OR BAD?

And the Lord spake unto Moses, saying, Speak unto the children of Israel, saying, Ye shall eat no manner of fat, of ox, or of sheep, or of goat. And the fat of the beast that dieth of itself, and the fat of that which is torn with beasts, may be used in any other use: but ye shall in no wise eat of it. (Leviticus 7:22-24)

The controversy continues to rage over fat – how much to eat, what kind to eat, etc. Man-made food rules seem to change weekly. Turn to God's Word. The instructions in Leviticus are clear – do not eat the fat of cattle, sheep, or goats. The fat being referred to is the cover fat of the animal rather than the fat that is marbled in the muscle tissue.

What makes the cover fat a problem for us? It contains higher amounts of toxins and contaminants than other tissue. Many people think that all toxins are eliminated by the body, but this is not the case. Various systems of an animal's body do attempt to remove toxic substances through eliminative channels; however, many toxins are simply stored. One of the major depositories is cover fat, which also happens to be high in saturated fats.

Notice that Holy Scripture does not advocate a no-fat or extremely low-fat diet. In fact, God's Word makes frequent reference to the consumption of olive oil and nuts, which are foods with high essential fatty acid content. Olive oil is high in monounsaturated fat, and those people in the Mediterranean areas who eat generous amounts of it have a very low rate of heart disease.

"Good" fats are critical to our good health. Dr. Nathan Pritikin, who advocated an extremely low-fat diet in order to protect himself from heart disease, died instead of leukemia. Scientific data has now shown us that extremely low fat consumption often leads to death from leukemia.

God calls us to balance, to moderation, to obedience, and to wise choices. In general, it is healthy to eat moderate amounts of fats found in the plant kingdom (such as nuts, seeds, grains, and natural oils) and small amounts of fat from the flesh of animals approved by God for food. Make no assumptions for your own particular situation, however. Ask the Holy Spirit to guide you in what is healthy for your body at this time.

Almighty God, I want to be aware of developing dietary information, but help me to overcome the temptation to act on it without first asking for Your guidance. Help me to choose healthy fats and healthy foods for the nourishment and healing of my body. Thank You for giving me the Holy Spirit who is my counselor and guide. I praise You, Father. In Jesus' name, I pray, Amen.

✝

DAY 36
WHAT ABOUT GRAIN?

Take thou also unto thee wheat, and barley, and beans, and lentils, and millet, and fitches [spelt], and put them in one vessel, and make thee bread thereof, according to the number of the days that thou shalt lie upon thy side, three hundred and ninety days shalt thou eat thereof.   (Ezekiel 4:9)

Or what man is there of you, whom if his son ask bread, will he give him a stone? Or if he ask a fish, will he give him a serpent?

If ye then, being evil, know how to give good gifts unto your children, how much more shall your Father which is in heaven give good things to them that ask him?   (Matthew 7:9-11)

Grains are one of God's special gifts. They can be cultivated all over the world under a wide variety of growing conditions, and they can be stored easily. Their diversity is amazing, ranging from wheat to corn to rice to rye to millet to oats and to quinoa. Almost every culture uses some form of grain as a staple in its diet.

Because bread was such an integral part of a healthy diet, Jesus used it to illustrate deeper spiritual truths. For example, He defined Himself as "the bread of life" (John 6:35) and, when He taught us to pray, He told us to say, "Give us this day our daily bread" (Matthew 6:11).

The bread of the Bible was very different from the bread we have today. The white bread which most people now eat has had most of its nutrients stripped from it during refining and processing, with only a few substances artificially replaced.

"Real" bread is dense, heavy bread made from whole grains. It is not loaded with preservatives and, therefore, spoils quickly if it is not refrigerated – hence, the phrase "give us this day our daily bread" has relevance at both the natural and spiritual levels of meaning. Bread made according to the recipe found in Ezekiel is now available commercially and provides a healthy option for bread in our diet.

In our "modern" times, people have developed various physical sensitivities to bread. One of the most common is gluten intolerance. One reason is that the necessary amino acids are no longer in the bread itself. Another is that many people's digestive tracts have been damaged and do not digest and assimilate all the components of bread properly. This is certainly not what God intended. He clearly intended for people to be able to eat wholesome bread and have it contribute to their good health.

Even if you have no gluten intolerance, eating excessive amounts of grains can make the body too acidic. Ask God what types of grains (and quantities) are healthy for you at the present time. You might also ask if Ezekiel's bread is right for you. Listen carefully and follow the guidance you are given.

Wonderful Father, thank You for grain and for giving me Your guidance about the healthiest way for me to include bread in my diet. *Thank You, God, for showing me the path to my healing. In Jesus' name, I pray, Amen.*

✝

DAY 37
NEW DISCOVERIES ABOUT WINE

And he will love thee, and bless thee, and multiply thee: he will also bless the fruit of thy womb, and the fruit of thy land, thy corn, and thy wine, and thine oil, the increase of thy kine, and the flocks of thy sheep, in the land which he sware unto thy fathers to give thee. (Deuteronomy 7:13)

... And Ziba said, The asses be for the king's household to ride on; and the bread and summer fruit for the young men to eat; and the wine, that such as be faint in the wilderness may drink. (2 Samuel 16:2)

The first miracle that Jesus performed was to change water into wine (John 2:7-11), and in the ordinance of the Last Supper He offered wine to His disciples as a symbol of the blood He was soon to shed for us (Matthew 26:28). We find numerous references in the Holy Scripture to the wise and moderate consumption of wine. Yes, we are talking about real wine.

Today there is much new research being done about a component of red wine called resveratrol, which appears to lower cholesterol and to inhibit certain cancerous tumors. Various studies have shown its effectiveness in dealing with colon, liver, and breast cancer. Thus far, it appears that resveratrol helps the cells to maintain healthy DNA and prevents cells from mutating into cancerous forms.

Red wine and grapes are high in antioxidants, particularly biologically active flavonoids. Flavonoids are effective in lowering LDL cholesterol, preventing arterio-sclerosis, and preventing blood clots.

The Holy Scripture is quite clear that the key to the consumption of wine is that it be done in moderation. Isaiah warns, "Woe unto them that rise up early in the morning, that they may follow strong drink; that continue until night, till wine inflame them!" (Isaiah 5:11). Isaiah reminds us that those people who consume alcohol of any kind are susceptible to spirits of addiction.

For those who would like the benefits of the grape and of red wine without the hazards and problems of alcohol, there is now an alcohol-free wine which is available. And resveratrol is also available in capsules.

Mighty God, today I give grateful thanks for the grape – and the many substances You placed in it for my nutrition, well being, and healing. Help me to use this fruit wisely in a positive, healthful way. As I add nutritious foods to my diet, I seek always to join with You in partnership for my recovery and healing. In the name of Your Son, Jesus Christ, my Savior and my Redeemer, I pray, Amen.

✝

DAY 38
THOSE PESKY DANDELIONS

O Lord, how manifold are thy works! in wisdom hast thou made them all: the earth is full of thy riches. (Psalm 104:24)

Have you ever bought some weed-killer to eliminate those pesky dandelions that pop up in your yard? The next time you see a lowly dandelion, think again, because it is a treasure-house of good nutrition and healing properties.

It is regrettable that we fail to educate ourselves about the riches of the earth and sources of good nutrition that exist around us. Think of the amount of money that is spent each year by people buying pesticides specifically to kill dandelions and in the process, poison the earth and water supply. Where yards have been sprayed with pesticides, the dandelions cannot be eaten for several years after the spraying has stopped.

It is quite likely that, if there are dandelions growing in your yard, you need them! The dandelion leaf has high levels of beta-carotene which provides a safe source of vitamin A for the body, and it is also a good source of potassium for muscular strength.

Dandelion leaves are beneficial to the skin and eyes, help keep organs free from mucus build-up and infection, strengthen the immune system, and assist those with low blood sugar to stabilize their blood sugar level. You can even put the lovely yellow flower petals in your salad for potassium, iron, and vitamin A.

Dandelion roots are a wonderful source of sodium, one of the primary minerals needed for the body to balance pH levels internally. Most people think of sodium in the form of salt or sodium chloride. It is very difficult for the human body to break the sodium chloride bond; consequently, there can be unhealthy complications from consuming large amounts of salt.

Interestingly, when you eat vegetable sources with high organic sodium content, you can actually drive out old inorganic sodium deposits from the body. Dandelion root extracts have historically been used for such health problems as muscle and joint stiffness, ulcers, stomach disorders, liver cleansing, and blood cleansing. It is a very valuable blood builder.

It is no accident that we have dandelions in our yards. They were put there in wisdom and were meant to be used for our nourishment and healing.

Almighty God, forgive me for being uninformed about Your creations. Forgive me for destroying what You created in wisdom. Help me to protect this earth and build my health. I want to learn, Father. In Jesus' name, I pray, Amen.

†

DAY 39
THE GOOD GIFT OF EGGS

If a son shall ask bread of any of you that is a father, will he give him a stone? or if he ask a fish, will he for a fish give him a serpent? or if he shall ask an egg, will he offer him a scorpion? If ye then, being evil, know how to give good gifts unto your children: how much more shall your heavenly Father give the Holy Spirit to them that ask him?   (Luke 11:11-13)

Controversy abounds about the advisability of eating eggs. One day the media reports on studies that warn us of the hazards from substances in eggs and another day the media reports on contradicting studies that report that eggs are good for us after all. For years we have been told that eggs were loaded with cholesterol and, therefore, we should avoid eating them. Then we were told that eggs also have high levels of lecithin which emulsifies cholesterol – so maybe eggs are not really so bad. In the confusion, we become more and more frustrated.

The egg is a very nutritious food. It is rich in essential fatty acids (especially omega 3), and half the fat in it is monounsaturated (like olive oil). Since it contains all eight essential amino acids, it is a very high-quality protein food. The problems appear to come when eggs are eaten in excess and when they are consumed in processed forms – such as powdered egg yolk. Also, hens are now caged, drugged with antibiotics, and generally live miserable, stressed lives. Therefore, we experience problems from eating the chemically-contaminated eggs laid by these hens.

The best way to cook eggs is to hard-boil them. Hardening of the arteries results from oxidized cholesterol, which is formed when you expose the egg yolk to air when you cook it, as in scrambling the egg. When you boil the egg, it is cooked without ever having air come in contact with the yolk. So you will be consuming cholesterol from the egg, but it won't be oxidized cholesterol.

The Holy Scripture offers basic guidelines for us. Jesus describes an organic, free-range egg as a "good gift" that a father would give his child. Jesus was the One who was sent to redeem us from our sins and our infirmities and to bear our diseases on the Cross. Surely He would not tell us to eat a food that would be universally harmful to our bodies. Of course, Jesus was talking about an organic egg coming from a free-range chicken who had *never* been given any chemicals of any kind – whether hormones or antibiotics or anything else.

God knows better than any person alive, better than any medical professional, better than any natural health advisor, better than any nutritionist, exactly what your particular nutritional needs are. Ask Him to reveal to you if you are to eat eggs. If you receive an affirmative answer, then ask for information on the precise quantity, frequency, cooking methods, and all the other details you need to know. Give grateful thanks to God for His guidance as you join with Him to restore your temple.

Wonderful Father God, thank You for the gift of the egg. Show me if I am to eat it at this time in my recovery. If so, teach me the ways to use it for my health and nutrition. In Jesus' name, I pray, Amen.

✝

DAY 40
WHY IS HYSSOP MENTIONED SO OFTEN?

Purge me with hyssop, and I shall be clean: wash me, and I shall be whiter than snow. (Psalm 51:7)

And the priest shall go forth out of the camp; and the priest shall look, and behold, if the plague of the leprosy be healed in the leper; Then shall the priest command to take for him that is to be cleansed two birds alive and clean, and cedarwood, and scarlet, and hyssop. (Leviticus 14:3-4)

Every time the Word of God mentions a food or an herb, we should let this spur our curiosity to see what its benefits are. It is interesting that hyssop is mentioned several times in the Bible. Let's take a look to see how it might be useful to us now.

Hyssop is most often mentioned in Scripture with regard to its cleansing function. Just as we were spiritually cleansed by the blood of Jesus when we were born again, we can experience physical cleansing internally to wash our bodies clean from toxins. Hyssop was widely used for that purpose in Biblical times, although other herbs are used more routinely today. Hyssop lubricates internal tissue fluids and removes debris from the surface of all body parts, such as the lungs, stomach, and blood vessels. This action results in great improvement of absorption and elimination.

When you feel sick, it may be appropriate to begin a program for cleansing. However, depending on your individual situation, you may need to build rather than to cleanse initially. When doing a cleansing, particular attention needs to be given to the colon, liver, and blood. There are many herbs and essential oils which have been used historically for their effectiveness and there are numerous preparations available. Ask the Holy Spirit what you need to do at this time and follow the guidance that you are given.

There are numerous additional functions for hyssop. Since it is an expectorant, hyssop has been used for generations for coughs, colds, asthma, and removing lung congestion. It has been used historically to improve sluggish circulation, aid digestion, expel gas, and promote sweating to reduce fevers. It may be useful for diseases affecting the skin, such as smallpox and chicken pox. Hyssop may be used externally as a poultice to help heal cuts and to relieve muscular rheumatism and bruises.

God provides us generously with herbs and essential oils that are to be used for maintaining and recovering our health. Learn about them and then ask the Holy Spirit to guide you as you seek your own recovery.

Father God, thank You for the abundance of herbs and essential oils which You have provided me. Show me teachers who can expand my knowledge of Your healing plants. Guide me through the Holy Spirit if You want me to do any internal cleansing at this time. In Jesus' name, I pray, Amen.

†

DAY 41
IS BUTTER GOOD FOR YOU?

Therefore the Lord himself shall give you a sign; Behold, a virgin shall conceive, and bear a son, and shall call his name Immanuel. Butter and honey shall he eat, that he may know to refuse the evil, and choose the good. (Isaiah 7:14-15)

Right here in the midst of a majestic passage about the coming of Jesus, the Holy Spirit talks about butter. Butter! This is a food that some authorities have told us is very unhealthy for us to eat. But Isaiah tells us that the Messiah will eat butter and honey. Why? So that He will know how to choose the good and to refuse the evil. Isn't that an interesting statement? Think about it for a moment and meditate on it.

Our health – or lack of it – is in large part due to the consequences of choices we have made. Years and years of unwise food consumption eventually take its toll on our organs, and we become ill. Certainly Isaiah is not suggesting a diet of nothing but butter and honey; however, he is clearly stating that butter and honey are classified as good things.

The latest scientific reports seem to be confirming Isaiah. We humans invented margarine with the intention that it be an improvement over natural butter, but now it appears that margarine creates health problems that are worse than the ones we thought butter caused.

Being a saturated fatty acid, butter does contain cholesterol. However, it is digested by the human body in such a way that generally does not raise the levels of harmful fats in the blood. Eaten in moderation, it is indeed a good food.

Remember, too, that the butter discussed in the Holy Scripture was made from wholesome, raw, organic milk from healthy animals. Amazingly, bacterial counts allowed today for raw milk are far lower than that for pasteurized milk, thus making certified raw milk cleaner than pasteurized milk.

Should you eat butter? Certainly stop eating margarine and fake, man-made substitutes. Go in prayer, ask the Holy Spirit what you should do and follow His advice. Maintain your health with wise food choices.

Wonderful Father God, too often I follow the opinions of men instead of asking You for guidance. Then when things go wrong, I turn to You. Help me, Lord, to go to You first. All I need to do is to take the time to ask, and yet I too often find excuses for not doing so. I want to manifest my healing, so instruct me about the foods that You want me to eat. Help me to work in full partnership with You, my God who heals me. In the name of Your Son, Jesus Christ, I pray, Amen.

SECTION THREE

HEALTHY EMOTIONS
FOR
HEALTHY LIVING

We are a three-part being – spirit, soul, and body.
Our spirit is saved and sealed by the Holy Spirit
when we give our lives to Jesus.
Our body is the physical house we walk in.
Our soul is made up of our mind, will, and emotions.
How we deal with emotions
has a critical effect on our health
and whether we live a healthy, vigorous life.

For more on this topic,
please read *The Power of God's Word
For Overcoming Hindrances to Healing, Volume 3*
where we discuss numerous ways
that emotions hinder the manifestation of healing.

†

DAY 42
LOVE IS ESSENTIAL FOR HEALING

Ye are my friends, if ye do whatsoever I command you. Henceforth I call you not servants; for the servant knoweth not what his lord doeth: but I have called you friends; for all things that I have heard of my Father I have made known unto you. Ye have not chosen me, but I have chosen you, and ordained you, that ye should go and bring forth fruit, and that your fruit should remain: that whatsoever ye shall ask of the Father in my name, he may give it you. These things I command you, that ye love one another. (John 15:14-17)

Repeatedly, Jesus exhorts and encourages every believer to follow through with His instructions. Notice that in this verse His instruction is a commandment, not a suggestion or an idea for us to consider. Jesus tells us that what He is saying is part of the "musts" of life. You must do what I am telling you if you want the result I promise, He declares. You have to do it this way. There are definite strings to the gift that is offered.

What is the command? Love. We know we feel love for certain people. But love as a feeling is weak because love is really action. It comes to life in what we do. And Jesus sets the standard very high by telling us we are to love everyone including our enemies.

Take some time to make an accounting of the ways that you demonstrate your love. Set aside a few minutes at the end of the day to list five ways that you put your love in action during the day. Maybe you prepared dinner for your family with a song in your heart and love flowing into the food instead of with complaints and pressure and unhappiness. Maybe you wrote a "thinking of you" card that you had put off for days. Maybe you spent some extra time brushing your pet and giving him attention.

If we want to fulfill our purpose, we have to get in the love business. Remember the incident when at the age of 12 Jesus had gotten separated from His earthly parents in Jerusalem and was found teaching in the synagogue? He told Mary and Joseph that He had to be about His Father's business.

Here He tells us that we are now in the Father's love business as well. Jesus has chosen us, and He has told us everything we need to know. It is up to us to respond to the call.

Gracious Father, thank You for the love You shower on me every minute of every day. I want to be about Your business of spreading Your Word and of being a living example of Your love to all who see me. Let me be a glorious example for others, manifesting my healing to Your glory. In the name of Your Son, Jesus Christ, Amen.

✝

Day 43
The Fruit Of The Spirit

But the fruit of the Spirit is love, joy, peace, longsuffering, gentleness, goodness, faith, meekness, temperance [self-control]. (Galatians 5:22-23)

While you need to be aware of your sins and of the ways you get out of agreement with God, it is more beneficial to keep your focus and attention on those things which bring you into alignment with God. These are the positive forces that make you strong spiritually, mentally, and physically and that fortify your shield of protection from the evil one.

Paul lists the fruit of the Spirit – love, joy, peace, patience, gentleness, goodness, faithfulness, meekness, and self-control. That's quite a list. When you feel sick, you need particularly to cultivate the fruits of positive qualities in your life and apply them not only to the people around you but also to yourself.

We often think it is selfish to be kind and gentle to ourselves. Yet Jesus plainly told us to love our neighbors as ourselves. Not more than or less than, but the same as. Frequently, one of the contributing causes to our illness has been our failure to treat ourselves lovingly and caringly. Applying the fruit of the Spirit is being self-full, not self-ish. It is part of fulfilling God's plan for us.

On this list of virtues, one of the major elements needed in recovery is self-control. God requires that you be a partner in your healing. That means that you need to be willing to make changes where you have gone astray. Do you want to be healed enough to do your own part? Or are you wishing to be well so that you can keep doing what you have always been doing?

Doing what you did got you where you are. Be willing to make changes in your prayer and meditation time, in your diet, in your physical activity level, and in your thinking patterns. Wellness is not just the absence of disease. It is a way of being. It is a way of living that allows God to work His will for you.

The fruits of the Spirit issue from a heart dedicated to the Lord. Turn every aspect of your life over to Him. Glorify Him in every action.

Loving Father, help me to stay focused on the fruits of the Spirit. Keep my eyes trained on You. Help me to fulfill Your will and Your purpose for me and to cultivate love, joy, peace, patience, kindness, goodness, faithfulness, gentleness, and self-control. In the name of Your Son, Jesus Christ, my Savior and my Redeemer, I pray, Amen.

✝

DAY 44
REJOICE EVERY DAY

This is the day which the Lord hath made; we will rejoice and be glad in it. (Psalm 118:24)

Every day when you first open your eyes in the morning, say, "This is the day which the Lord has made. I will rejoice and be glad in it." Fill your heart and soul with these words, and each cell in your body will receive the message, too.

Life is a gift, and the Word says God wants you to have so many days that they will add up to a very long life. You can pick up the daily newspaper and read item after item from the front page to the back page about people for whom today did not come. If they died before fulfilling the long life promised by the Father, then the enemy stole their time.

What if you have felt sick for a long time? What if you are in discomfort or pain? What if the night has seemed very long and all the medical reports are grim and you really want an end to it all? When this is how you feel, "rejoicing and being glad in the day" seems beyond comprehension.

Your answers can be supplied only by God. Immerse yourself in Holy Scripture so that you can find faith to hold onto. "For I know the thoughts that I think toward you, saith the Lord, thoughts of peace, and not of evil, to give you an expected end [a future and a hope]" (Jeremiah 29:11). "I am the Lord that healeth thee" (Exodus 15:26). "For with God all things are possible" (Mark 10:27).

Select the passages that speak to you and put them on a note card beside your bed. When you wake up in the morning, read each verse and then say, "God, I stand on Your Word. You have a purpose for my life and You have made every provision for me. I receive the healing You have provided through the atonement of Jesus on the Cross. This is the day which You have made. I will rejoice and be glad in it." After you do this for a few days, you will be surprised at the difference you will begin to notice in yourself.

Spend time every day taking note of the things for which you can rejoice and be glad. No matter what your situation is, there are things worthy of thanksgiving. Focus on those. Rest in the Lord and praise His name.

Merciful God, there are times when I struggle and when I feel overwhelmed by the symptoms of my illness and by the appearance of my situation. Give me courage to see Your truth beyond the circumstances that surround me. I am filled with Your strength and grace. Let me rise up every morning declaring, "This is the day that You have made and I do rejoice in it." Thank You, Father, for healing me. In the name of Your Son, Jesus Christ, my Savior and my Redeemer, I pray, Amen.

✝

Day 45
The Healing Power Of Music

Let the word of Christ dwell in you richly in all wisdom; teaching and admonishing one another in psalms and hymns and spiritual songs, singing with grace in your hearts to the Lord.
(Colossians 3:16)

One of the best ways to promote your healing is to fill your life with music. Paul very wisely exhorted the Colossians to sing "psalms and hymns, and spiritual songs." Interestingly, he told them something even more important – something about their attitude. They were to sing with grace in their hearts to God.

When you feel discouraged or are in pain or just feel out of sorts with your life, few things can restore you more quickly than music that fills your soul. Create a library of hymns and songs of praise and worship which bring joy to your heart and peace to your soul. Make listening to these praise songs a part of your daily activities. Play them while you are in the car or doing household chores. In some cases, it is feasible to play them as background music while you are working; you may be surprised to find that you accomplish your tasks much more quickly and efficiently.

The more you listen, the more the message penetrates within. The vibrations of the sound waves actually create healthy vibrations within the cells of your body. Every organ and every gland get a little energy boost from the music and facilitate your healing. The words and the music join to create a unique method for healing. Think of every song as a healing treatment.

Join in with the music and sing along. Do not judge your musical ability. Just let go and sing. When you do so, breathe deeply from your abdomen and let your lungs expand. Feel your vocal cords vibrate and then feel that vibration resonate in every cell of your body.

Let your whole body become an instrument glorifying the Lord your Creator. Sometimes you may become so attuned that tears of joy suddenly start to flow as you are overwhelmed by the grace and love that surround you and fill you. Allow the Holy Spirit to speak to you and to bring you into deeper worship of the Father.

These moments are special gifts. Treasure them. Go in song to God often with gratitude on your lips and in your heart.

Gracious Father, I am delighted to be able to worship You with psalms and hymns and songs. Music fills me with a feeling of awe and joy and vitality. It renews my mind and bolsters my faith. I sing my praise to You, Father. In the name of Christ Jesus, my Savior and my Redeemer, I pray, Amen.

†

DAY 46
SINGING SONGS OF GRATITUDE

Sing, O heavens; and be joyful, O earth; and break forth into singing, O mountains: for the Lord hath comforted his people, and will have mercy upon his afflicted. (Isaiah 49:13)

Over and over again, we are taught the connection between expressions of joy and our healing. Here in Isaiah we have a beautiful poetic verse: "Sing, O heavens; and be joyful, O earth; and break forth into singing, O mountains: for the Lord hath comforted his people, and will have mercy upon his afflicted."

How can you put this part of God's Word into effect in your life? First, think of something in your life for which you are especially grateful. Think of how blessed you are to have this person or thing or situation in your life. Now say out loud, "Thank you, God for _____!" Keep saying "thank you" out loud. As you focus on your thankfulness more and more, do you sense a deep joy rising up inside of you?

Now find some exuberant music filled with praise and worship for the Lord. Sing along with all your heart as the music energizes you. Your blood and lymphatic circulation increases, and your breathing becomes more rapid. More healing oxygen and nutrients get to your cells.

Next, it is time to make a different selection of music. Select songs that are filled with tranquil worship, songs that tell the story of God's love and compassion, of His strength and His power, of His wondrous grace. Let the music and the words cradle your soul and heal your body. As you listen, climb into the lap of your Heavenly Father, just as a little child goes to a loving parent. Feel how soothing and gentle His touch is.

How often do you experience this comforting touch of God? It may be that the answer is "not often." If that is the case, you need to realize that Jesus asked Father God to give you the most incredible gift of all, the perpetual presence of the Holy Spirit within you. Every born-again believer has the guarantee of the comfort of God through the blood of Jesus. Allow the Holy Spirit to comfort you day by day, hour by hour, minute by minute, and second by second.

Whether you "feel" Him or not, the Holy Spirit always abides with you and in you. He never leaves you and is always present to guide and to comfort you. Rest in Him with songs of thanksgiving.

O merciful Father, joyful, joyful, I do adore You. I sing with the heavens and with the earth in praising You for Your comfort and Your mercy. You sent Your Word and healed me, and You still shower me with blessings. In Jesus' name, I pray, Amen.

✝

DAY 47
LIVING IN JOY HELPS TO HEAL YOU

A cheerful look brings joy to the heart, and good news gives health to the bones. (*Proverbs 15:30 New International Version*)

Laughter heals. Smiling heals. Joy heals. It is almost impossible to recover from illness if you spend all your time bemoaning your aches and pains and making every detail of the recovery process a chore and a burden.

Yes, there is a time for serious attention to the steps you must take. But overall, you must learn to lighten up and to approach each day with cheerfulness and with joy in your heart. Too many of us think that Jesus was somber and serious all the time. Listen to these words: "These things have I spoken unto you, that my joy might remain in you, and that your joy might be full" (John 15:11). Jesus speaks of joy, both His joy and our joy.

Just for a moment close your eyes and imagine Jesus standing before you. See Him step close and then see His eyes light up with delight. His mouth turns up into a big smile and then He breaks out into laughter. He speaks your name and says, "Share my joy. Laugh with me." And He laughs some more.

Smile. Laugh. Join Jesus in laughter. Throw your arms up into the air and skip around like a little child for no reason other than the most glorious one of all: you are loved with an everlasting love by the ever-faithful Father and by His Son Jesus Christ.

Take your most troublesome problems and give them to your loving Savior. Feel the lightness, the joy, and the laughter that fills you as relief floods your being.

How important it is to have a heart filled with joy! "This is the day which the Lord hath made; we will rejoice and be glad in it" (Psalm 118:24). Sing your praise! Laugh your praise! Smile your praise! What a wonderful way to witness to others by showing them your life filled with joy and gratitude for your living God.

When you know you are walking according to God's will, you not only have peace in your heart but you also have laughter in your spirit and a smile on your face.

Father God, it is Your joy that fills me, and it is Your good news that gives health to my bones. I have many blessings for which to rejoice. My cup truly runneth over. You are my mighty protector and Healer. I sing before You, and I seek to radiate to all who see me the joy of my faith and trust in You. Thank You, Father, for loving me, for saving me, and for healing me. In the name of Your Son, Jesus Christ, I pray, Amen.

✝

DAY 48
JOY BRINGS HEALTH

All the days of the oppressed are wretched, but the cheerful heart has a continual feast. (Proverbs 15:15   New International Version)

Joy in your body brings health. Sadness, despair, and depression do not. It can be hard to be cheerful when you feel sick, but the paradox is that the more you focus on gladness, the more you create an internal environment for healing.

This concept was popularized most spectacularly by Norman Cousins who became very ill with a collagen disease in the mid-1960s. Even though he was in constant pain, he used laughter to stimulate his healing. He found movies, jokes, and stories that were funny, hilarious, and just plain silly. The more he laughed, the less pain he felt. Ten minutes of belly laughter produced two hours of sleep without pain. Hours of laughter each day produced more and more healing in his body which was repeatedly confirmed by laboratory tests.

When he had succumbed to the oppression of the disease, Cousins felt wretched. When he developed a cheerful heart, he found he had a continual feast of gradually improving recovery. And remember, he accomplished this all in the physical and soulish realm.

As a believer, you can apply these techniques in a much more powerful way by operating in the joy of the Lord. Adding the spiritual power and truth of the Word of God to the physical and soulish realms makes an unbeatable combination.

How much do you laugh during the day? Do you take your life and your illness or injury so seriously that there is no room for joy to fill you? Make a list of the things that make you laugh the deep-down, roll-on-the-floor belly laugh humor that is so funny to you that you laugh until tears roll down your cheeks. That is the laughter of healing.

Create your own "Laugh for Health" collection. Ask your friends and family members to send you clippings or jokes to add to your collection and to give you fresh material.

Make a commitment to spend time every day immersed in humor and in laughter. Make a joyful noise to the Lord. Come before Him with gladness.

Thank You, God, for the healing power of a cheerful heart. I choose to see the humor in every situation and to smile and laugh more often with my family and friends. Holy Spirit, fill me with Your joy so that I may experience every day Your healing laughter. The joy of the Lord is indeed my strength, and I laugh, Father, in sheer delight of Your goodness and mercy. In Jesus' name, I pray, Amen.

✝

DAY 49
THE HEALING POWER OF LAUGHTER

Then was our mouth filled with laughter, and our tongue with singing: then said they among the heathen [nations], The Lord hath done great things for them. The Lord hath done great things for us; whereof we are glad. (Psalm 126:2-3)

Because laughter is so healing, we are going to stay on this topic a little longer. When you laugh, physiological changes occur in the body, promoting healing in every cell in your body. Your pituitary gland releases substances called endorphins, which have a pain-relief action that is very strong. With intense laughter, tears can even stream from your eyes, giving them a cleansing bath.

Muscles in your head and abdomen contract, and your lower jaw actually vibrates. Your arteries tense and then relax. Your vocal cords contract making the music of laughter that can vary from loud guffaws to soft titters to an up-and-down roller coaster.

Your heart rate increases, and the extra blood flow sends more oxygen to all the cells of your body. Your lungs expand and your diaphragm is activated. Your nervous system triggers your adrenal glands to release adrenaline, which raises your energy level and lifts your spirits. Your leg muscles relax, and, if you laugh hard enough, you end up sitting down because you are literally too weak to stand.

Laughter has been described as "internal jogging" because it is so beneficial to all the organs, glands, and cells of the body. In the previous devotion, we learned how Norman Cousins actually created a healing program of laughter after developing a debilitating collagen disease. In case after case, people with arthritis, depression, and numerous other diseases have been helped tremendously by the simple act of laughing throughout their day.

No matter how serious the health challenge before you, remember the truth that the Lord God Almighty loves you and wants you well. Remember that nothing is too hard for God. Remember that no power (and that includes satan) is stronger than Jehovah-Rapha, the God who heals you.

Accept these truths totally, and you will be filled with praise which naturally bubbles out in the form of joy. And joy turns into laughter. Declare like the Psalmist, "The Lord has done great things for me, my mouth is filled with laughter, and my tongue is filled with singing."

Wonderful Father, thank You for the miracle of laughter. Thank You for all the healing actions it has in my body. Help me to see the humor in my life and to spend time every day laughing out loud and singing songs of joy. Father, you have done many great things for me, and I am filled with gratitude, happiness, and joy. Thank You for healing me. In the name of Your Son, Jesus Christ, I pray, Amen.

✝

DAY 50
THE BENEFITS OF SELF-DISCIPLINE

He will die for lack of discipline, led astray by his own great folly.
(Proverbs 5:23 New International Version)

Self-discipline is a major issue in healing and recovery from illness. There are many things that we know we should do, and we struggle to find the time to do them. Then on the other hand, there are many things that we know we should not do, and yet time after time we find ourselves doing them. The worst part is that we judge ourselves by our failures and then use our failing as an excuse to give up.

If you are having these problems, take a deep breath and know that you are under attack from the enemy. First, stop condemning yourself and lighten up. Smile. And begin again.

Suppose your eyes were attacked and you were guided by the Holy Spirit to provide extra nutrition for them with an herbal eyewash. You managed to do it for about a week, but then your schedule got crowded, your energy sagged, and you felt too irritable to do it.

Take your authority given in Luke 10:19 over every attack of the enemy. Then go in prayer to God, repenting for letting your struggles and your difficulties sidetrack you. Check with Him to make sure that you are still to continue the eyewash and to be clear about the particular herbs to use. Once you are certain about God's guidance, ask for help in making this part of your healing a priority in your life.

Spend some time in meditation to see if there are any spiritual blocks to your being healed. In this example, is there anything in your life – past, present, or future – that you don't want to see? Ask God to reveal to you what you need to know in order to allow you to receive the healing that is constantly flowing to you.

Then make a commitment to God to exercise self-discipline. Do not allow the evil one to sabotage your healing and lead you down the road of folly.

Enforce your authority, activate the power of God working through you, and offer each step in your program to God. Do everything in His name and for His glory.

Wonderful Father God, I do not want to die for lack of discipline, led astray by the evil one and my own great folly. Help me to be obedient and to offer every part of my healing program to You. I perform each act in Your name and for Your glory. I am determined to walk the path to my healing that You want me to follow. Thank You for leading me every step of the way. In the name of Your Son, Jesus Christ, I pray, Amen.

†

DAY 51
DON'T BE STUCK IN THE PAST

And Jesus said unto him, No man, having put his hand to the plough, and looking back, is fit for the kingdom of God. (Luke 9:62)

Not as though I had already attained, either were already perfect: but I follow after, if that I may apprehend that for which also I am apprehended of Christ Jesus. Brethren, I count not myself to have apprehended: but this one thing I do, forgetting those things which are behind, and reaching forth unto those things which are before, I press toward the mark for the prize of the high calling of God in Christ Jesus. (Philippians 3:12-14)

Too many of us waste our lives living in the past. We are consumed by resentment for wrongs done to us, by grief over losses and traumas, and by regret for mistakes and errors. We live with the words "if only" on our lips and spend endless hours reliving events that have long since passed.

This kind of behavior is fertile ground for the evil one. He loves to keep us mired in unresolved issues of the past because it is one of the best ways to prevent us from engaging in living in the present. We cannot be here, fully present today in our body and soul, when we are focused on yesterday. If we are constantly looking behind us, we can't see where we are, and we will drive blindly into the future.

The failure to connect with the current moment creates a spiritual imbalance that leads to a mental and physiological imbalance. Illness often results.

Are you living in the past? Write down issues that concern something that happened in the past but still occupy your attention. Ask for forgiveness for your part in those events. If you need to make atonement to someone, do it.

It is likely that some of the items on your list may be deliverance issues. Examples are grief that lasts for years and years, resentment that has a stranglehold on your relationships, or rage that repeatedly explodes on a moment's notice. The Lord has provided complete deliverance so that you will be free to move on!

Paul says that he forgets what is behind and instead takes hold of Christ Jesus. Today is all we really have. Yesterday is gone. And tomorrow is always a day away. Christ Jesus offers us life abundant today, this moment. Live in Him and glorify His name.

Father God, I let go of the past and connect fully to You in this glorious day that You have given me. Forgetting what is behind, I press on in Your service, standing on Your Word and following Your Son, Jesus Christ. In Jesus' name, I pray, Amen.

†

Day 52
Create A Bible Study Group
For Healing

And let us consider how we may spur one another on toward love and good deeds. Let us not give up meeting together, as some are in the habit of doing, but let us encourage one another – and all the more as you see the Day approaching. (Hebrews 10:24-25 New International Version)

We have seen the huge proliferation of support groups that have sprung up for people who have specific illnesses and diseases. People go for emotional support, for information, and for advice. These groups are generally secular in nature and are centered around agreement in certain conventional medical treatment. As a general rule, they are not very open to exploring alternative methods of healing.

What we must never forget is that the Word of God has to be the central focus and the central guideline for every single thing that we do. Therefore, you may wish to start a special Bible study group for people who are being attacked with illness. This Bible study would first and foremost be centered on worship of the Lord God Almighty and His Son, Jesus Christ. It would be a place where people come to spur one another on, provide encouragement, and dig deep into the Word to shine the light of truth, thus destroying all the lies of the enemy.

There can be a short portion of time in each meeting set aside for the sharing of information and ideas, not only about conventional treatment possibilities but also on the numerous natural treatment methods. This is a time to glorify the God of all creation and to examine His provision for us through His plants and natural remedies.

There is a real danger, however, that the enemy will try to make these suggestions the focus of the meeting, so set a timer if necessary to control the length of time spent concentrating on medical and herbal suggestions rather than the finished work of the Cross. It is also important to remember that members of this group will need to be willing to look at the spiritual causes of their illness and to join together in the process of repentance and deliverance.

The primary focus of the group should always be this: *What does the Word of God say* about healing, about deliverance, about recovery, and about being made whole? Our own ideas are not important. What is important is what *God* says about the matter. And then it is up to each one of us to get into agreement with God. If that means that we change our mind and re-evaluate our beliefs, then so be it.

We need each other. We need to pray with and for each other. Jesus told us that where two or more were gathered, He would be in their midst. Where else would Jesus want more to be than in the midst of those earnestly seeking liberty from their infirmities? Join together to proclaim that by His stripes we are healed.

Father God, help me to find other people who will stand with me on Your Holy Word that by the stripes of Jesus we are healed. I want support from others who keep me focused on Your Word and who encourage me to strengthen my faith by calling things that are not as though they were. What a joy it is to have special people to pray with me and to walk in victory with You. In the name of Your Son, Jesus Christ, I pray, Amen.

✝

DAY 53
HAVE THE ATTITUDE OF GRATITUDE

By him therefore let us offer the sacrifice of praise to God continually, that is, the fruit of our lips giving thanks to his name. (Hebrews 13:15)

Like a child who flings his arms around the neck of a loving parent with an exuberant hug, we run to God with prayers of gratitude, saying, "Thank You, thank You, thank You!" The writer of Hebrews reminds us to say "thank You" continually, which means to keep on doing something without stopping. Amazing! We are to say "thank You" constantly in songs of praise. Why? Because every good gift comes from God and the least we can do is to be grateful.

An attitude of gratitude is vital for those who feel ill because the easier path is often to be critical and hard to please. It is tempting to give in to depression, listlessness, and crankiness. These are attacks from the enemy and if you allow yourself to spin in negative thoughts, you are giving the evil one a dangerous foothold in your soul and body. As a result, you will probably find your illness penetrating even more deeply.

Post little note cards in the rooms of your home. All they have to say is "Say thank you." Be sure to put two or three in your kitchen. Put one on your refrigerator and one on your kitchen cabinet where you keep your dishes.

Why is the kitchen important? Because nutrition provides the building blocks at the physical level for you to heal. Saturating your food in generous amounts of gratitude will have a positive effect in the way you digest your meals and in the way you assimilate the nutrients.

What a difference gratitude makes! Saying "thank You, thank You, thank You" a hundred times a day brings the healing power of love into your body. Gratitude can actually create a change in your body chemistry, transforming every cell.

As you reach up to God with thanksgiving, He smiles down on you with His healing grace. The "You're welcome" of God and the Holy Spirit is a shower of healing water that purifies you and washes you clean.

Wonderful Father God, thank You, thank You, thank You. Every minute of the day is a gift from You. I joyfully sing my praises of thanksgiving, and I declare my gratitude for the many blessings You shower upon me. I choose to be positive. I choose to focus on Your goodness and mercy. I choose to maintain an attitude of gratitude. And I choose to look up and glorify You. In the name of Your Son, Jesus Christ, my Savior and my Redeemer, I pray, Amen.

†

DAY 54
THANKSGIVING IS
YOUR GOD-CONNECTION

Enter into his gates with thanksgiving, and into his courts with praise: be thankful unto him, and bless his name. (Psalm 100:4)

O give thanks unto the Lord, for he is good: for his mercy endureth for ever. ... Oh that men would praise the Lord for his goodness, and for his wonderful works to the children of men! And let them sacrifice the sacrifices of thanksgiving, and declare his works with rejoicing. (Psalm 107:1, 21-22)

Rejoice evermore. Pray without ceasing. In every thing give thanks: for this is the will of God in Christ Jesus concerning you. (1 Thessalonians 5:16-18)

Thanksgiving, praise, and rejoicing are at the heart of worship. Each of these elements builds on each other and provides a way to strengthen your relationship with God. When you offer your thanks to Father God, you draw close to Him in love and adoration. He has given us every good and perfect gift and is worthy to be praised and glorified.

Notice how often praise and giving thanks are linked in Scripture. They go hand in hand because they keep us focused on the good things that God has given us. They lead us to enumerating all the blessings that are flowing to us and do not allow us to think about our problems or our difficulties.

Notice that Paul connects rejoicing, prayer, and thanksgiving. He exhorts the Thessalonians to give thanks in everything, in all circumstances. You are not giving thanks *for* your illness but *despite* your illness. No matter how bad things look, you can always find something worthy of gratitude.

The evil one wants you to focus on the negative, including all the things that you have done wrong and all the mistakes that you have made. He wants you to focus on your weaknesses, your failures, your inadequacies, your aches and pains, and medical predictions of gloom.

Do not allow satan to take control over you or your thoughts. Christ Jesus defeated the evil one and rose victorious. Stand up in your faith, and exercise the power that was won for you.

Join the hosts of heaven in singing, "Blessing, and honour, and glory, and power, be unto Him that sitteth upon the throne, and unto the Lamb for ever and ever" (Revelation 5:13).

Father God, thank You, thank You, thank You. I joyfully give thanks for Your many blessings and for Your constant love. I worship You, Father, and with deepest gratitude thank You for the victory of the finished work of the Cross. In the name of Your Son, Jesus Christ, I pray, Amen.

†

DAY 55
YOUR NEED FOR PEACE

And let the peace (soul harmony which comes) from Christ rule (act as umpire continually) in your hearts [deciding and settling with finality all questions that arise in your minds, in that peaceful state] to which as [members of Christ's] one body you were also called [to live]. And be thankful (appreciative), [giving praise to God always].   (Colossians 3:15   Amplified Bible)

Is your heart filled with peace and soul-harmony? Peace is a pool of tranquility that reflects your connection to the Lord. It is one of the things that people value most and yet rarely have.

There is no peace if we are filled with bitterness about our health condition. There is no peace if we are filled with loneliness and despair. There is no peace if we are angry with our family and friends. There is no peace if we are terrified about our future. There is no peace if we are afraid to die. And there is no peace if we are afraid to *live*.

The expansion of this Scripture that is provided by the Amplified Bible helps us to understand the intent of Paul's words. He so beautifully explains how it is that we can have peace in our hearts. It is through letting Christ and the Holy Spirit rule in our hearts and settle with finality all questions that arise in our minds. All questions!

When we feel sick, there are many decisions to be made and the choices seem endless. If we use our own wisdom or that of other people only, we are often burdened with doubts about whether we have done the "right" thing or the "wrong" thing.

Instead of struggling with these decisions, we need to turn them over to God and let Christ rule in our hearts. We are then guided to the right path for us, and the result is peace in our soul. We are called to *live*, not merely to survive in a desperate struggle from one day to the next.

Take your concerns to God in prayer now and then listen for the Holy Spirit to speak to you. Receive the peace of Christ and give thanks.

Gracious God, sometimes I am tempted to let myself be overwhelmed and caught in a trap of confusion. I take captive every thought of doubt and unbelief and renew my mind instead with Your Word. I choose to let the peace from Christ rule in my heart and settle with finality all my questions and concerns. I joyously proclaim Your truth that by the stripes of Jesus I am healed. I give You glory and praise and honor, Father. Rule my heart, rule my life, and direct my path so that I can glorify Your Holy name. In Jesus' name, I pray, Amen.

SECTION FOUR

SPIRITUAL GUIDELINES FOR HEALTHY LIVING

God's Word has much to say
about developing a strong spirit
in order to fulfill God's plan for our lives
in a healthy, courageous way.

✝

DAY 56
IMMERSE YOURSELF IN GOD'S WORD

He sent his word, and healed them, and delivered them from their destructions. Oh that men would praise the Lord for his goodness, and for his wonderful works to the children of men! And let them sacrifice the sacrifices of thanksgiving, and declare his works with rejoicing. (Psalm 107:20-22)

... quicken thou me according to thy word. ... This is my comfort in my affliction: for thy word hath quickened me. (Psalm 119:25, 50)

God's Word in the Holy Scripture is inspired by the Holy Spirit, and it shows you God's overall plan for you as His beloved child. It reveals to you how God works in your life and how God wants you to act and to live. It contains God's promises to you as well as God's commands.

Immerse yourself in God's Word, and ask the Holy Spirit to reveal to you particular passages that are most relevant for you for that day. Holy Scripture is meant to lift you up, to strengthen you, and to bring you into closer communion with the Lord God Almighty. "To quicken" means to be made alive, so Holy Scriptures are meant to make you more alive and more vibrant in your service to God. The Psalmist says, "Revive me, and make me alive and vibrant according to Your Word, God. This is my comfort in my affliction, for Your Word has given me life."

155

God has declared Himself as Jehovah-Rapha – the God who heals us (Exodus 15:26). This name establishes God's covenant with us. It does not speak only of God's promise to us, but it shows us who He really is. God is our Healer. He sent His Word and, therefore, sent His healing. It is done. It means little to believe that God *can* heal someone else unless you believe that God is healing *you*.

God's Word is not just in the form of the Holy Scriptures, but it is also in the person of His Son, Jesus Christ. God "sent His Word and healed them," Psalm 107 verse 20 says. Believe that God's Word and God's Son were sent for you personally. Scripture says that "God anointed Jesus of Nazareth with the Holy Ghost and with power: who went about doing good, and healing all that were oppressed of the devil; for God was with him" (Acts 10:38). God's Word says that "with His stripes we are healed" (Isaiah 53:5).

So, stand on the Word of God and receive your healing.

Almighty God, You have named Yourself as Jehovah-Rapha, the God who heals me. You sent Your Word both as Your Son and as Holy Scripture to heal and deliver me from my destruction. I praise You for Your goodness and for Your wonderful works. I rejoice and give You thanks. I receive Your healing, and I praise Your Holy name. Thank You for making me alive and vibrant according to Your Word. In Jesus' name, I pray, Amen.

†

DAY 57
MAKE TIME FOR GOD'S WORD

So then faith cometh by hearing, and hearing by the word of God.
(Romans 10:17)

My soul melteth for heaviness: strengthen thou me according unto
thy word.   (Psalm 119:28)

For this cause also thank we God without ceasing, because, when
ye received the word of God which ye heard of us, ye received it not
as the word of men, but as it is in truth, the word of God, which
effectually worketh also in you that believe.
(1 Thessalonians 2:13)

Faith comes by hearing, and hearing by the Word of God. If we want to develop our faith, we must immerse ourselves in God's Word and absorb it into our mind and heart. This requires a commitment of time on a daily basis so that we may be filled at every level of our being with God's glorious good news.

Examine the habits of your life. Do you find ways to integrate God's Word into your daily living patterns? There are several simple techniques to do this.

For example, each week select a particular verse of Scripture that uplifts you and write it on a couple of note cards. Then post these note cards in places where you will see them frequently – on the refrigerator door or the bathroom mirror or the television remote control! Every time your eyes see the card, make sure that you read the message with intent and focus.

Another way to incorporate the Word into your life is to get CDs or downloads of the Psalms or the New Testament or the entire Bible. Play these recordings in the car while you are commuting to work, running errands, or driving children to their activities. Listen while you are taking a walk or doing your exercise. You will be surprised at how much "Word" time you will have.

When the Word is a part of you, then it can work effectively in you and through you so that you will be a glorious witness to others.

Wonderful Father God, thank You for Your Holy Word, which strengthens, supports, and encourages me. As I hear Your voice, I step out in faith. Reveal to me creative ways to make time for filling my mind and heart with Holy Scripture. Let Your Word work effectually in me, and let me be a joyous witness of Your love and care and healing power. In the name of Your Son, Jesus Christ, I pray, Amen.

†

DAY 58
MAKE AN INVENTORY
OF THE BENEFITS OF SICKNESS

For I came down from heaven, not to do mine own will, but the will of him that sent me.   (John 6:38)

Healing has to be the will of God because Jesus tells us clearly that He came to do only the will of our Heavenly Father.   Ordained at the time of Adam and Eve's transgression, Jesus' purpose was prophesied by Isaiah. Jesus was sent by the Lord God Almighty to redeem our sins, bear our infirmities on the Cross, and heal everyone who came to Him.

It is Jesus' desire to heal because He always works the Father's will. Before He healed a crippled man, Jesus asked Him, "Will you be made whole? Do you want to get well?" (John 5:6). What is your response? Before you blurt out a "yes," imagine for a moment the full implication of your answer.

Infirmities often provide a hiding place for us. When we feel sick, we frequently do not have to take full responsibility for the details of life. Other people sometimes give us more attention and support when we feel ill than they do when we are well. We even can get away with being irritable and difficult, letting our buried anger bubble out over those around us.

Take time to make a full internal inventory. Do it on paper by writing down all the disadvantages of feeling sick. That is the easy part and your answers will probably come quickly. Now write down the benefits you receive by being ill – those quiet, subtle things that hide, protect, and shield you from engaging fully with life and with other people. Give yourself several days to do this. Pray to the Holy Spirit to reveal to you what you need to know. If you feel bold, ask a trusted friend to help you.

Once you have both lists, decide whether you are willing to give them to God. You cannot give up one list and keep the other. You either relinquish them both or hold onto them both.

If you are sure you are ready to give them to your Heavenly Father, ask for forgiveness for allowing these things to take control of your life. Humble yourself before God with a repentant heart, and ask Him to cleanse you in mind, soul, and body. Sometimes when these items represent major strongholds of the enemy, you may need to seek out spirit-filled believers to help you take authority in order to be set totally free.

Stand on the Word that it is God's will for you to be made whole and well.

Gracious God, Jesus said that He came down from heaven not to do His own will, but to do Your will. Everywhere in the Gospels it is recorded that Jesus healed everyone who came to Him for healing. No one was turned away. And Your Word says that by His stripes I was healed because Jesus took my sicknesses for me. I stand in faith, Father, and I declare that by His stripes I was healed. In Jesus' name, I pray, Amen.

✝

DAY 59
WORSHIP THE LORD

But the hour cometh, and now is, when the true worshippers shall worship the Father in spirit and in truth: for the Father seeketh such to worship him. God is a Spirit: and they that worship him must worship him in spirit and in truth. (John 4:23-24)

The four and twenty elders fall down before him that sat on the throne, and worship him that liveth for ever and ever, and cast their crowns before the throne, saying, Thou art worthy, O Lord, to receive glory and honour and power: for thou hast created all things, and for thy pleasure they are and were created. (Revelation 4:10-11)

And every creature which is in heaven, and on the earth, and under the earth, and such as are in the sea, and all that are in them, heard I saying, Blessing, and honour, and glory, and power, be unto him that sitteth upon the throne, and unto the Lamb for ever and ever. (Revelation 5:13)

Communion with God is found in worship. Jesus tells us that Father God is a spirit and that we must worship Him in spirit and in truth. The core of our relationship is worship – glorifying the Father, praising the Son, and communing with the Holy Spirit.

Worship is the most profound when it is the most simple. We proclaim the honor and power of our God and our Savior. We keep our thoughts focused on His majesty,

His power, and His love. We lose ourselves in Him, acknowledging His abiding presence with us every moment of the day and night. For those who have been baptized with the Holy Spirit, this is a wonderful time to pray in tongues as Paul says in 1 Corinthians 14:2.

When we feel sick, it is sometimes easy to become so focused on the healing that we want to see manifested that we spend more time telling God about our situation than we do in pure worship. While worshipping, we are not asking for anything at all. It is a time to glorify and magnify our Father who so loves us that He sent His Son to save, heal, deliver, and make us whole. It is a time to praise and honor Jesus Christ who paid every price in full for us.

Make sure that you have time set aside in your day for pure worship.

Father God, You are worthy to receive glory and honor and power because You have created all things. I am awed that Your Word says that You created me for Your pleasure. Blessing and honor and glory and power be to You that sits on the throne and to the Lamb forever and ever. In Jesus' name, I pray, Amen.

✝

DAY 60
LET SPIRITUAL MENTORS LIFT YOU

And the servant of the Lord must not strive; but be gentle unto all men, apt to teach, patient, in meekness instructing those that oppose themselves; if God peradventure will give them repentance to the acknowledging of the truth; And that they may recover themselves out of the snare of the devil, who are taken captive by him at his will. (2 Timothy 2:24-26)

Do you have any spiritual mentors? God meant for us to have guidance at the earthly level to help us as we grow spiritually, to provide a spiritual "covering," and to keep us on the right track. It is important that you have some spiritual mentors and that they walk in the revelation knowledge of salvation, healing, deliverance, and being made whole.

What should the primary characteristics of your counselors be? Since we are going to be divulging our deepest, most vulnerable self, we need people who have a great capacity for tenderness. Paul lists gentleness, patience, and meekness. It is important that we be treated kindly and with respect, just as Christ Himself treats us with the greatest love.

What is it that these spiritual leaders do? Paul tells us that they instruct "those that oppose themselves." Isn't that an interesting way to describe the times when we are our own worst enemy? God is always for us. It is satan who seeks to get us to oppose ourselves and to harm ourselves. And how does satan do that? By bringing us into captivity.

Our spiritual teachers point out the places where they see that we have allowed satan to gain a foothold. Then they make every effort to help us to acknowledge the truth and to bring us to repentance. Why? So that we "may recover ourselves (and come to our senses) out of the snare of the devil." Caught by satan, we have been taken captive and are now following him and doing his will instead of following God and doing His will. Our teachers will be able to help us be set free so that we can be restored to freedom and wholeness.

Strong spiritual teachers and counselors are vital to the mental, spiritual, and physical health of each one of us. Your pastor is your earthly spiritual head and should be your primary spiritual leader. Ask God to direct you in finding others to help you grow in spiritual wisdom and strength.

Almighty Father, I need strong spiritual counselors in my life because I know there are many times when I oppose myself. Lead me to Your servants who can gently and patiently instruct me, assist me in acknowledging Your truth, and bring me to repentance so that I can recover myself, come to my senses, and be set free from the snare of the devil. I want to do only Your will, Father. Only Yours. In Jesus' name, I pray, Amen.

†

DAY 61
CELEBRATE COMMUNION

That the Lord Jesus the same night in which he was betrayed took bread: And when he had given thanks, he brake it, and said, Take, eat: this is my body, which is broken for you: this do in remembrance of me.

After the same manner also he took the cup, when he had supped, saying, This cup is the new testament in my blood: this do ye, as oft as ye drink it, in remembrance of me. For as often as ye eat this bread, and drink this cup, ye do show the Lord's death till he come.

Wherefore whosoever shall eat this bread, and drink this cup of the Lord, unworthily, shall be guilty of the body and blood of the Lord. But let a man examine himself, and so let him eat of that bread, and drink of that cup. For he that eateth and drinketh unworthily, eateth and drinketh damnation to himself, not discerning the Lord's body. For this cause many are weak and sickly among you, and many sleep.   (1 Corinthians 11:23-30)

Celebrating communion on a daily basis is a powerful way to bring an awareness of the resurrection power of Jesus to your remembrance. Paul says that we can take the Lord's Supper as often as we like, so why not incorporate it into your worship?

Each time you receive the elements, you speak God's victory into your body and soul. By the stripes of Jesus I am healed, so I eat this bread to remind myself that the beaten, broken body of Jesus paid for my healing. Through the blood of Jesus my sins are forgiven, so I drink this cup to remind myself that the shed blood of Jesus purchased complete salvation for me, including healing, deliverance, and being made whole.

Paul gives a warning to the Corinthians about taking the Lord's Supper carelessly or irreverently. Many of you are sick and weak and in fact many have died, Paul says, because you are being careless by taking communion without regarding the finished work of the Cross properly. It is up to you to reject all carnal things that turn you away from the spiritual walk. Make sure you aren't harboring unforgiveness in your heart toward anyone. Examine yourself and judge yourself, he pleads.

Communion joins us together in a precious moment of worship. Even when we are taking communion alone at home, we know that believers all over the world share this sacred sacrament with us. Examine yourself and receive the bread and the cup in memory of the victory of the Cross.

Father God, I forgive those who have offended me and all those against whom I have harbored resentment. I take the bread and the cup in awe of the supreme sacrifice and great victory won for me by the stripes and the blood of my Savior, Jesus Christ in whose name I pray, Amen.

†

Day 62
What Is Being Carnally-Minded?

For to be carnally minded is death; but to be spiritually minded is life and peace. Because the carnal mind is enmity against God: for it is not subject to the law of God, neither indeed can be. So then they that are in the flesh cannot please God. (Romans 8:6-8)

This is a hard Word. "They that are in the flesh cannot please God." Paul is teaching us the tough truth that we cannot stay focused on carnal, bodily, earthly things because all those things lead to death.

"The carnal mind is enmity against God: for it is not subject to the law of God, neither indeed can be." Paul is talking about our soulish realm which is our mind, our thoughts, our emotions. Our natural mind is an enemy of God and at war with Him. Why would Paul say that? Because our mind did not get saved at the moment of salvation. Our spirit did and is sealed forever by the Holy Spirit.

As we know, we have to renew our mind constantly. We say that statement fairly easily, but when it comes down to the specifics of what that means, we often rebel. Are you really willing to look at all the carnal, worldly things that you fill your mind with?

For example, how much television do you watch? And what kind of shows do you enjoy? Do you fill your mind with shows that glorify killings and adultery and sexuality? Don't deceive yourself that it isn't affecting you because it is. Whatever God calls an abomination is "enmity against Him." You cannot associate with it and think you can go untouched.

Television. Movies. Dirty jokes. Vulgar speech. The list is long of worldly things that are enemies of God. Removing yourself from things that are not pleasing to God gets hard to do. Your carnal self will protest. "But can't I have any fun?" "But all my friends like to put a couple of bucks on our poker game. It's just for fun."

If you allow mixture in your life, you are yielding yourself to the enemy. And every time you yield, you create hindrances to your receiving your healing. You are no longer single-minded, and you are voluntarily giving the enemy authority in your life. You can't stand against the enemy in one area so you can be healed and yet invite him in in another area so you can have a temporary moment of "fun."

God exhorts you to be spiritually-minded and to have life abundant.

Father God, there are areas in my life where I have been carnally-minded. I don't want to have parts of myself in opposition to You, Father. Give me courage to examine my life carefully and root out all influences that are not pleasing to You. In the name of Jesus, I pray, Amen.

✝

DAY 63
HOW SOWING AND REAPING AFFECT YOUR HEALTH

Be not deceived; God is not mocked: for whatsoever a man soweth, that shall he also reap. (Galatians 6:7)

God has established several spiritual laws, and one of the most important is that what we sow determines what we reap. Whatever we do has effects and consequences. The interesting thing is that for the most part these consequences are not unexpected. Yet time and again we claim surprise because we want to blame someone or something other than ourselves for the situation in which we find ourselves.

If you want to be well, you must understand this principle. God will not be mocked. You cannot violate His laws of good health and then moan and pretend to be innocent. If you poison the soil with chemicals and spray your food with pesticides, you can expect to reap the deadly results. If you sit all day and don't move your body, you can expect to reap the crippling results. If you stress yourself by working at a job that is not God's plan for you and that you do not love, then you can expect to reap the depleting results.

You reap not only what you sow yourself, but you also reap what your parents and your grandparents have sown.

At the physical level, as each generation does things which weakens them, they pass along DNA that is a little weaker to each succeeding generation.

God has given us authority to have dominion here on earth. We forget this fact and instead blame God in times of disaster and hold Him responsible for making us sick. "It's God's will," we claim. We fail to look at all the ways that the seeds of illness were sown by us and our parents and do not want to accept the responsibility of reaping the consequences.

If we have made bad choices, there is a way that we can have a fresh beginning – by truly repenting. Through the atonement of the Cross Jesus has provided that your sins be forgiven, your deliverance accomplished, and your body healed and made whole.

God loves you. You are important to Him because, as a born-again believer, you are His child. He forgives you of your sins, and He heals you of your diseases. He has given you every tool so that you can walk in victory.

Dear God, I know I am reaping what I have sown. I am truly sorry for the mistakes that I have made that have contributed to my current health situation. Having repented of my sins, I am taking action to live differently. Thank You for wiping the slate clean so that I can plant new seeds and reap a harvest of health and wholeness. Thank You for Your miraculous restoration of every cell in my body and for healing me through the stripes of Jesus. In Jesus' name, I pray, Amen.

✝

Day 64
How To Pray For Healing

...The effectual fervent prayer of a righteous man availeth much.
(James 5:16)

We want our prayers to "avail much," but exactly how do we pray effectively for our healing? First, acknowledge the sovereignty of God, who has made us so awesomely.

Second, affirm your belief that Jesus carried to the Cross not only your sins but also the particular health condition that you have named. Jesus has already released you, and it is extremely important that you claim His victory. Third, look for the spiritual roots of the health problem you are having. Repent of your sins and ask forgiveness.

Fourth, thank God for sending His Word and healing you. Ask for the manifestation of healing for your particular health condition if you have never asked for it previously. If you have already asked, you do not need to ask again. Praying isn't begging, whimpering, and pleading repeatedly for the same thing. Instead, trust that you have been heard, and offer continual prayers of thanksgiving.

Fifth, enforce God's Word on your body, and speak with authority to the parts which are out of balance. Command every cell, gland, and organ to operate perfectly.

And cast every lying symptom out of every cell of your body. Whenever symptoms appear, use Luke 10:19-20 and Mark 11:23-24 as your guidelines, and command the enemy to leave.

Sixth, ask for God's guidance for any steps you need to take in order to facilitate your healing. Ask Him to reveal to you the things you need to do in the natural realm to support your body in repairing and rebuilding itself.

Last, declare your belief in your healing. Confess over and over again that God's healing power is at work in your body. Believe before you see. Do not make the mistake of basing your belief on what you see in the natural world. Stand on God's Word. Speak God's Word numerous times during the day.

Almighty God, Your Word tells me that great power is released when I come to You in prayer. How grateful I am that You are my God who is approachable, who knows me by name, and who cares about me personally. I release all those who have hurt me, and I forgive each one. Forgive me, Father, for carrying resentment, anger, and unbelief. In the name of Your Son, Jesus, I command every lying symptom of the enemy to leave me, and I command every cell, tissue, organ, and gland to function perfectly. Heavenly Father, show me anything You want me to do to assist my full recovery and to maintain my good health. Thank you for healing my body, my mind, and every part of me. In Jesus' name, I pray, Amen.

†

Day 65
Be Still Before The Lord

Be still, and know that I am God. (Psalm 46:10)

Everyone needs focused time with God. For most people this takes the form of prayer, which is a vital part of our spiritual life. It is a time for us to tell our Father how much we love Him and how grateful we are for His many blessings. It is a time for us to intercede for others. And it is also a time for us to share all the things on our heart.

However, when we pray, we are busy talking to God and are not allowing Him any opportunity to speak to us. Hearing God's voice is critical because we can't align ourselves with God's will for us if we do not listen to Him. It is interesting that most of us were taught as children to pray, but few of us were taught to listen to the Lord.

Most people find it difficult to "find the time" to listen to God. They may say their morning or evening prayers and some find time for daily reading of Holy Scripture. But quiet, focused listening is rare. Why is that? Perhaps it is due to the fact that we are often afraid of what we will hear. There isn't much point in taking the time to listen to God, if we do not intend to act on the guidance that we are given. But to do so often takes great trust and boldness because sometimes God's guidance does not seem logical or realistic and sometimes it differs from the opinions of people we trust.

Turn to God's Word. The Bible is filled with accounts of people who listened, who heard, and who acted. Often, they endured great ridicule when they did so. Can you really imagine what Noah went through while he was building the ark?

Get still in your mind. Begin to talk to God and the Holy Spirit. Do not spend time detailing your ailments. God already knows your problems, and He has already provided the solution through the finished work of the Cross. Talk to Father God with the easy conversation that you would have with your best friend. Ask any specific questions that you may have. And, in the name of Jesus, muzzle every voice from the enemy that will try to distract you or tell you lies.

Then be still in the presence of the Most High God. Just be still. Experience the peace that passes all understanding. Rest in the Lord and He will speak to you. He is ever-faithful to guide with His loving hand.

Father God, I set aside all the voices of my family, friends, and advisors and open my heart to You. I've listened to their opinions, but now I want to hear only Your voice, Father. I still my mind. I will act on Your guidance and follow Your direction for my life. And now I will be silent and listen, Lord. I will be silent and listen. In Jesus' name, I pray, Amen.

†

DAY 66
MAKE EVERY ACT A PRAYER

And whatsoever ye do in word or deed, do all in the name of the Lord Jesus, giving thanks to God and the Father by him. (Colossians 3:17)

If your healing comes instantaneously, praise God! That is God's best. However, if the manifestation comes gradually, there is no condemnation for being on a slower path to victory.

There are many things you can do to promote your recovery, but be aware that the evil one wants to sabotage your healing and will throw up obstacle after obstacle to your recovery program. There will be many temptations to stop or change your course. Life itself will get in the way. Even friends and family may get in the way.

How do you maintain the self-discipline to do what you need to do? Follow God's instructions and dedicate every small action to the Lord. "Whatever you do in word or deed, do it all in the name of the Lord Jesus, giving thanks to God." That means that everything you do becomes a prayer.

Every herb you swallow for the health of your liver is a prayer. Every step in a walk you take for the strengthening of your heart is a prayer. Every essential oil you apply for the perfect function of your joints is a prayer. Every weight you lift for the strengthening of your bones is a prayer. Every vegetable you eat for the nourishment of your body is a prayer.

Pray while you are doing whatever you are doing. Thank God over and over again for your healing. Praise Him. Glorify Him. You may find that you begin to look forward to tasks that were once a chore. You sing and hum and pray while you are doing them, and they don't seem to take as long. You realize that, as you are glorifying God, you are celebrating your healing and are being revitalized.

A prayer is no longer just something you say; it is living praise to God as you carry out His will in your life.

Wonderful Father God, whatever I do, whether in word or deed, I do it all in the name of the Lord Jesus. I give thanks to You, Father, and I am so grateful for Your constant love and guidance. I am awed by the sacrifice that was made for me on the Cross. My sins and all my infirmities were overcome there. I am saved. I am redeemed. I am healed. Show me what You want me to do to support my health and wholeness. Your will be done on earth, Father, as it is in heaven. I am Your instrument in Your service. In humble gratitude I pray in the mighty name of Jesus, my Lord and Savior, Amen.

✝

Day 67
Praying In Faith

Be not rash with thy mouth, and let not thine heart be hasty to utter any thing before God: for God is in heaven, and thou upon earth: therefore let thy words be few.   (Ecclesiastes 5:2)

But when ye pray, use not vain repetitions, as the heathen do: for they think that they shall be heard for their much speaking. Be not ye therefore like unto them: for your Father knoweth what things ye have need of, before ye ask him.   (Matthew 6:7-8)

Jesus tells you not to turn your prayers into a kind of mindless chant, saying the same thing over and over. Instead, "let your words be few." He is telling us not to babble on and on and on, but to get right to the point with God. Why is succinct prayer important? Because prayer is communion with God. Through your prayers, you reflect the type of relationship you have with your Heavenly Father.

Both the words you use and the style of your speech reflect the quality of your faith. If you keep going on and on, wallowing in your problem, you exhibit a lack of faith that Father God is your healer. If you pray over and over for healing, you prove either that you do not believe you have been heard or that you do not believe God has already taken action in your behalf through the finished work of the Cross.

For example, suppose a friend asks for a loan and you tell him that you will give it to him at the end of the week when you get paid. If your friend doubts you, he will keep asking you about the loan. If he trusts you, he will say nothing more until he receives the money.

So what is the best way to pray for healing? Jesus asked the blind man, "What do you want me to do?" (Luke 18:41). Tell Jesus just once what you want. Then you enforce the Word. In the name of Jesus bind every spirit of infirmity that is attacking you. Call things that be not as though they were and command your body to be healthy in the name of Jesus.

Most important, thank and praise God constantly that He has healed you. Speak the Word often, declaring that by the stripes of Jesus you are healed. Proclaim loudly that Jesus took your infirmities and bore your sicknesses. Stand firm on God's Word and actively enforce it on your body.

Dear Father, I speak to You from my heart, simply and without pointless repetitions. I love walking with You in sweet communion as a child walks with a loving parent. You already know every need I have, so I choose to rest in Your peace and love and grace. Nothing will shake my faith, Father, that Your Word is true and that Jesus is my Risen Lord, who has purchased my healing for me through the stripes He took and His shed blood. In Jesus' name, I pray, Amen.

✝

DAY 68
DO YOU KNOW
WHAT GODLY MEDITATION IS?

When I remember thee upon my bed, and meditate on thee in the night watches. (Psalm 63:6)

I will meditate also of all thy work, and talk of thy doings. (Psalm 77:12)

My hands also will I lift up unto thy commandments, which I have loved; and I will meditate in thy statutes. (Psalm 119:48)

... but I will meditate in thy precepts. (Psalm 119:78)

Mine eyes prevent the night watches, that I might meditate in thy word. (Psalm 119:148).

Till I come, give attendance to reading, to exhortation, to doctrine. ... Meditate upon these things; give thyself wholly to them; that thy profiting may appear to all. (1 Timothy 4:13, 15)

It is well known in the secular and medical world that meditation is beneficial to people, both emotionally and physically. Numerous types of meditation classes can be found, including transcendental meditation and yoga, and sadly many churches even offer these courses. The basic technique is to make your mind "blank," especially by repeating a sound like "Ommm" endlessly.

Beware of this kind of meditation (no matter what name is used for the class). The blunt truth is that it is a form of New-Age philosophy, and the forces of the enemy are behind it. Meditation is never meant to be a "zoning out" into mindlessness in which the mind thinks nothing. Here is the reason why it is so dangerous. The enemy loves an empty mind because that allows him to move in and take control. The visions and images and "truths" that come from such practices are not godly because their source is the enemy. Do not be deceived. Mindless meditation provides an open door for the enemy to move in and take control.

What are the Biblical standards for meditation? Look at the Scriptures above and notice the profound difference between secular/eastern meditation versus the kind of meditation that God tells us to do. God's Word speaks often of meditation, but here is the critical point you must understand. Meditation is *always* meditating on God, His Word, or His work. Let me repeat that statement. Meditation is *always* meditating on God, His Word, or His work. Meditation is never, ever mindless. It always, always, always keeps your mind full to the brim with Him – which is the exact opposite of emptying your mind and thus inviting the evil one to come in.

In meditation we fill our mind with the Word and then simply stop speaking in order to let the Holy Spirit speak to us. Quietness is not mindlessness. In quietness we open ourselves to revelation directly from the Holy Spirit, and we are enveloped with the peace of God.

Father God, let the words of my mouth and the meditation of my heart be acceptable in Your sight, O Lord, my strength and my Redeemer. Forgive me for participating in mindless meditation and deliver me from any demonic spirits that I allowed into my mind by engaging in that activity. I will never practice mindless meditation again, Father, but will focus on You, Your Word, and Your mighty work. It is my desire that I always stay full of You in my mind, my thoughts, my emotions, my body, and my spirit. In Jesus' name, I pray, Amen.

✝

Day 69
Keep A Journal Of God's Actions In Your Life

I will meditate on all your works and consider all your mighty deeds. (Psalm 77:12 New International Version)

Bless the Lord, O my soul: and all that is within me, bless his holy name. Bless the Lord, O my soul, and forget not all his benefits: who forgiveth all thine iniquities; who healeth all thy diseases; who redeemeth thy life from destruction; who crowneth thee with lovingkindness and tender mercies; who satisfieth thy mouth with good things; so that thy youth is renewed like the eagle's. (Psalm 103:1-5)

What wise advice to meditate on all the mighty works of the Lord God Almighty in your life! You are exhorted to "forget not all his benefits." Take a moment to assess your words and thoughts yesterday. Did you spend more time praising God for His mighty deeds in your behalf, or did you spend more time focusing on your problems and deficits and needs?

For the next week, make a commitment to yourself to keep a journal of all the mighty deeds of the Lord acting in your life. Remember that every positive event in your life is a mighty deed, so don't discount anything, no matter how small it might appear to you.

For example, suppose you were able to slice a tomato without pain in your hands. Praise God and put it on your list. Or maybe you received a note from a friend. Or a little bird perched on a branch outside your window and sang a song to you. Maybe the sunset was especially beautiful. Or it rained. Or it snowed.

Praise and thanksgiving to the Lord changes our focus. God's Word clearly tells us that the important things are the things of the spirit which cannot be seen with our human eyes. We have to be so convinced of this truth that no doubts creep in and no unbelief causes us to waver in our thinking.

It's very beneficial to spend time at the end of each day to review your list of the mighty deeds of God. Give grateful thanks for each item. Tell the Lord how much you love Him and worship Him and trust Him. Thank Him for forgiving all your sins and healing all your diseases.

Let His joy fill you and His peace sustain you.

Wonderful Father God, I come to You with a grateful heart, and I praise Your Holy name. I am awed by the mighty deeds that You are working in my life. All that is within me sings to You, O Heavenly Father, "Thank You, thank You, thank You!" For Yours is the kingdom and the power and the glory. In Jesus' name, I pray, Amen.

†

DAY 70
WAIT UPON THE LORD

But they that wait upon the Lord shall renew their strength; they shall mount up with wings as eagles; they shall run, and not be weary; and they shall walk, and not faint.   (Isaiah 40:31)

Out of God's love for us, He offers His strength, His power, and His healing. These magnificent benefits flow from Him constantly, as He is always present to lift us up and keep us going forward.

Take a few minutes to meditate on this verse and imprint its meaning in your heart. Allow its truth and power to take hold in your soul and body.

As you do this exercise, you may or may not "feel" the presence of God. We know that the Word of God tells us that the Holy Spirit resides in every born-again believer. So even though faith is not based on feelings, there can be a tangible, positive "feeling" of the presence of God when we place ourselves in a focused attitude of worship.

But before you begin, please do not fall into the deception that you have to "feel" God's presence in order to believe that He is with you. And do not chase after these feelings by thinking that you have not "really" worshipped unless you have "felt" God's presence with your physical senses.

Begin by getting your Bible, settling into a comfortable chair, and relaxing. If you have some quiet, inspiring worship songs, play them now. Open your heart and soul to God and worship Him in the spirit. If the Holy Spirit brings particular Scriptures to mind in addition to this passage from Isaiah, look them up and meditate on the messages being revealed to you.

Now in your mind's eye, see yourself as God sees you through the blood of Jesus – totally well. See every cell and every organ in your body working to perfection. In particular, see the part of your body that satan has attacked as healthy and strong. See yourself serving God in vigor, in joy, and in humility. Ask God to show you the purpose He has for you to fulfill.

Declare yourself strong, vigorous, and running the good race for the Lord. Thank your Heavenly Father that you are able to serve Him and glorify His name.

Loving Heavenly Father, thank You that my strength is renewed. I declare that I soar on wings like eagles, that I run and am not weary, that I walk and do not faint. I rely on You totally for my strength and energy to continue in my recovery and to keep moving forward in service to You. I refuse to accept any lying symptom in my body, and I declare boldly that by the stripes of Jesus I was healed and am healed. I am so grateful that Jesus took every one of my infirmities and bore them away so that I don't have to endure them. Thank You, Father; thank You. In Jesus' name, I pray, Amen.

✝

DAY 71
SPEAK THE WORD AND HOLD ON

Seeing then that we have a great high priest, that is passed into the heavens, Jesus the Son of God, let us hold fast our profession. (Hebrews 4:14)

The writer of Hebrews encourages us to "hold fast our profession." Our profession of faith is our confession of what we believe. It consists of our words. What we say is critical because all of creation began with God's Words. The Almighty *spoke* us into being.

Then He instructed us to do the same thing. For example, Moses was to *speak* to the rock to get it to produce water (Numbers 20:7-12). Joshua was to *shout* and the walls would come tumbling down (Joshua 6:15-20). Other actions and works would follow, but *first* was the spoken word.

Jesus continued the example of His Father by *speaking* to the wind and the waves to quieten them. He *spoke* to disease, and it left people's bodies. He *spoke* to dead bodies, and they were filled with life once more. Mighty and glorious works followed after the proclamation of the Word.

It is vital that we do the same thing. So, speak to your illness and infirmity, and enforce God's Word on it. Speak to the enemy and command every spirit of infirmity to leave

189

you. Command every organ and cell in your body to function perfectly according to God's design. Quote your favorite healing Scriptures over your body and your life. Say out loud, "By His stripes I was healed. Himself took my infirmities and bore my sicknesses."

Now that you have spoken your confession of faith, you have to "hold fast" to it. Jesus always kept His mission clearly focused in His mind and heart, and He held fast to His purpose without ever wavering. Do you profess Jesus Christ as your Lord and Savior? Then hold fast to His instruction in the Great Commission to "observe all things whatsoever I have commanded you" (Matthew 28:20).

Do you profess Jesus Christ as the one who "took our infirmities, and bare our sicknesses" (Matthew 8:17)? Then hold fast to the fact that this includes you. Jesus Christ your Savior took your infirmities and carried your sicknesses to the Cross. Profess this belief and hold fast to it.

Do you profess the promise of Jesus who said "if you abide in me, and my words abide in you, ye shall ask what you will, and it shall be done unto you" (John 15:7)? Then do as your Savior instructs. Live in Him, walk according to God's will, and hold fast to the promise of your healing.

Do you profess Jesus Christ who said, "Verily, verily, I say unto you, He that believeth on me, the works that I do shall he do also; and greater works than these shall he do; because I go unto my Father" (John 14:12)? Then let every thought and every action fulfill His words and hold fast to your trust that Jesus spoke the truth.

It is easy to say words, to make a verbal profession of belief. The hard part is to live the words you speak. Holding fast is faith in action. It is belief manifested by doing. Hold fast to the promise of your healing. Hold fast to God's Holy Word. Hold fast to your belief that satan has been defeated. Hold fast to the sovereignty of the Lord God Almighty.

Father God, I profess my faith that You are the God who heals me. I profess my faith in Your Son, Jesus Christ, who took my sins and infirmities to the Cross. I hold fast, I look past my symptoms, and I focus on Your healing power. You are my deliverer, protector, and healer. Thank You, Father. I know that I am Your beloved child and that You hold me in the palm of Your hand. I dwell in the secure knowledge that all victory is mine by the promise of Your Holy Word. In the name of Your Son, Jesus Christ, I pray, Amen.

✝

DAY 72
TALK TO YOUR BODY

... For this purpose the Son of God was manifested, that he might destroy the works of the devil. (1 John 3:8)

Just exactly what were the works of the devil that Jesus destroyed? The Word is full of examples. If the devil had attacked people with illness in their bodies, Jesus healed them. If the devil had led them into prostitution, He provided deliverance and told them to go and sin no more. If the devil had made them mentally ill, He healed their minds. If the devil had convinced them to steal from others, He healed their soul and led them to repentance and atonement.

Again and again and again, Jesus set people free. As Acts 10:38 tells us, He "went about doing good, and healing all that were oppressed of the devil."

Have no doubt that the source of illness is the devil. If you feel sick, satan has a foothold in your body. Luke 10:19 gives you power "over all the power of the enemy" so enforce that power over the attack of the devil. Speak with authority to satan and to your illness. Command the devil to leave in the name of Jesus Christ, who defeated satan forever.

Enforce the Word of God on him and on the illness that is present. Follow the example of the Lord God Almighty and of Jesus Christ and speak God's truth into being.

Talk to the cells that are malfunctioning and tell them to resume normal activity. Talk to the organs of your body and tell them to stabilize and perform their functions according to the divine plan of the Almighty. Over and over again, confess your belief that the healing power of God is working mightily in your body.

Name each system of your body – immune, digestive, intestinal, nervous, glandular, endocrine, urinary, skeletal, muscular, reproductive, respiratory, sensory, and circulatory – and command each one to be made whole in the name of Jesus Christ. Command each body system to function normally according to its divine purpose.

Confess over and over again that by the stripes of Jesus you were healed. And finally repeat healing Scriptures aloud because doing so will help to build your faith and keep it strong. Jesus has won the victory for you, so rejoice!

Almighty God. I enforce Your Word on every cell in my body. By the authority of Luke 10:19 and in the name of Your Son, Christ Jesus, I command every spirit of infirmity to leave my body. I command every cell, every gland, every organ, and every system to function normally. I rejoice in my healing, Father, and receive it now. In the mighty name of Jesus, my Lord and Savior, I pray, Amen.

✝

DAY 73
THE POWER OF YOUR OWN WORDS

Pleasant words are as an honeycomb, sweet to the soul, and health to the bones. (Proverbs 16:24)

Words have great power. God's Holy Word is the ultimate Word and the ultimate power. Jesus Himself embodied the Word: "In the beginning was the Word, and the Word was with God, and the Word was God" (John 1:1).

Jesus told us how important words are because they reveal our inner condition and reflect what we are thinking and what we are feeling inside. It is not the things that we eat that make us either clean or unclean "but those things which proceed out of the mouth [that] come forth from the heart" (Matthew 15:18).

Pleasant words, positive words, agreeable words all affect us. They are "sweet to the soul" because they put us in greater harmony with our God of love and compassion and kindness. They bring us closer to Him. Each word is a seed, and pleasant words will bear sweet fruit.

This verse in Proverbs reminds us that positive thoughts and words have a major impact on our health. They are "health to the bones" which is a way to describe health all the way through our body to our innermost core. Words are understood by the cells in our body, and these cells take our words literally, just as we think or say them.

For example, when we use expressions such as "I'd die for a soft drink!" or "That joke just kills me!" our body takes the words at face value. When we say, "I am a diabetic" or "I have heart disease," our body actually works to fulfill the meaning of those words.

Be mindful of your words today, both spoken and unspoken. Let them be positive words that agree with the Word of God. If negative words pop out, say immediately, "Cancel that," and then make a positive statement instead.

Continue developing this habit until you have transformed your speech and your thoughts. This brings you into partnership with God, pleases Him, and removes hindrances to your healing.

The Lord has given us every tool we need so that we can receive everything He died to give us. The table is prepared before us and on it is salvation, healing, deliverance, and being made whole. Reach out and take everything you desire.

Heavenly Father, today I will be mindful of every word I think and every word I say. I know the power of words, and I seek to use that power for Your glory, for the benefit of others, and for my own good. I affirm Your Word which declares, "I am the God who heals thee." I proclaim the Word of Jesus Christ who said, "Your faith has made you well." Today I will let the words of my mouth and the meditations of my heart be positive, uplifting, and acceptable in Thy sight. I choose to receive everything that Jesus died to give me. I give you all the glory and all the praise and all the thanks for my salvation, healing, deliverance, and being made totally whole. In the name of Your Son, Jesus Christ, my Savior and my Redeemer, Amen.

✝

GREAT RESOURCES

Our YouTube Channel

Youtube.com/c/ProclaimingGodsWord
Be uplifted and encouraged by tranquil, inspirational videos with Scripture and music on topics such as healing, peaceful sleep, and overcoming depression.

Books and Teaching CDs

1) *Sparkling Gems from the Greek, Vol 1*
2) *Sparkling Gems from the Greek, Vol 2*
3) *Paid in Full, An In-Depth Look at the Defining Moments of Christ's Passion*
4) *A Light in Darkness*
5) *No Room for Compromise*
By Rick Renner
Renner Ministries
P.O. Box 702040, Tulsa, OK 74170-2040
918-496-3213
renner.org

1) *Dismantling Mammon*
2) *Healed: Once And For All*
3) *No More Curse*
4) *Releasing Seed That Produces Kingdom Dominion*
5) *Pressed Beyond Measure*
6) *Freedom Through the Anointing*
7) *Victory – What Would You Do If You Knew You Could Not Fail?*

By Pastor Tracy Harris
Harvest International Ministries
4000 Arkansas Boulevard
Texarkana, AR 71854
870-774-4446
experiencehim.org

1) *Authority of a Renewed Mind*
2) *Preparations for a Move of God*
3) *The Spirit of Elijah is in the Land*
4) *Hope for the Heart*
5) *Your Robe of Righteousness*
6) *Proving God*
7) *The Healing Library*

By Dr. Sandra Kennedy
Sandra Kennedy Ministries
2621 Washington Road, Augusta, GA 30904
706-737-4530
sandrakennedy.org

1) *You've Already Got It*
2) *Believer's Authority*
3) *A Better Way to Pray*
4) *The True Nature of God*
By Andrew Wommack
Andrew Wommack Ministries
P.O. Box 3333, Colorado Springs, CO   80934-3333
719-635-1111
awmi.net

1) *Atonement*
2) *You Shall Receive Power*
3) *Blessing or Curse*
4) *The Basics of Deliverance*
By Derek Prince
Derek Prince Ministries
P.O. Box 19501, Charlotte, North Carolina 28219
704-357-3556
derekprince.org

1) *The Tongue – A Creative Force*
2) *Can Your Faith Fail?*
By Charles Capps
P.O. Box 69, England, AR 72046
501-842-2576
charlescapps.org

The Living Christ in You
By James W. Gardner
P.O. Box 2127, Jasper, AL 35502
205-221-1747
jasperchristiancenter.org

Christ the Healer
By F. F. Bosworth
1973, Fleming H. Revell, division of Baker Book House Co.

How to Live and Not Die
By Norvel Hayes
Norvel Hayes Ministries
P.O. Box 1379, Cleveland, TN   37364
423-476-1018

Music – Online, Downloads, CDs

soulkeeperradio.com
Soulkeeper Radio. Streaming peaceful Christian music that will restore, renew, and refresh your soul. While you are working on your computer, have soothing Christian music playing. This is a very special website, run by Melissa and Joe Champlion.

Audiobooks For *The Power of God's Word*

Audiobooks of *The Power of God's Word* are available at Amazon.com, iTunes.com, and Audible.com.

Books by Anne B. Buchanan

From God's Heart to Mine
This is a blank journal for recording the words that God speaks to you. There is a special foreword explaining the purpose and power of keeping this journal.
Available at Amazon.com

Christian Devotional Healing Series
If you like this book from *The Power of God's Word* Christian Devotional Healing Series, then you will love the other volumes.

Get the series:

- From Amazon.com.
- Audiobooks from Amazon.com and Audible.com.

Volume 1 – *The Power of God's Word for Healing*
70 daily devotions! You will learn:

- Why misunderstanding what the word "saved" means can keep you from being healed.
- Why saying sentences with "I am" can either help you recover or keep you sick.
- Why there is power for healing in communion.
- Why your words determine your health.
- And much more!

<u>Volume 2 – *The Power of God's Word for Receiving Healing*</u>
65 daily devotions! You will learn:

- Why it is critical to know the difference between facts and the truth.
- Why the unbelief of others can affect your recovery.
- How to look beyond the appearance of your ailments.
- Why not consulting God first can trap you.

<u>Volume 3 – *The Power of God's Word for Overcoming Hindrances to Healing*</u>
78 daily devotions! You will learn:

- Why misunderstanding Job will keep you sick.
- Why Paul's thorn was not sickness.
- Why suffering sickness does not glorify God.
- Why it is almost impossible to be healed if you don't do three important things.
- How to pray effective prayers instead of prayers that actually hinder your recovery.

<u>Volume 4 – *The Power of God's Word for Healthy Living*</u>
73 daily devotions! You will learn:

- Five easy habits to develop to promote your health.
- Why herbs and essential oils are God's blessings for healing.
- Three emotions that are critical for good health.
- Why it matters what music you listen to.
- Why some kinds of meditation hurt you instead of helping you.

A Final Word

I pray that you have been encouraged, lifted, and inspired by these devotions. May you walk in victory and divine health.

If you like this book, I would really appreciate your leaving a review for it at Amazon.com. It would be a blessing for me, and I would be very grateful.

End Notes

Cover photograph by Philippe Put
    www.flickr.com
    License: Attribution 2.0 Generic (CC BY 2.0)

97032472R00115